THE

NORDIC

WAY

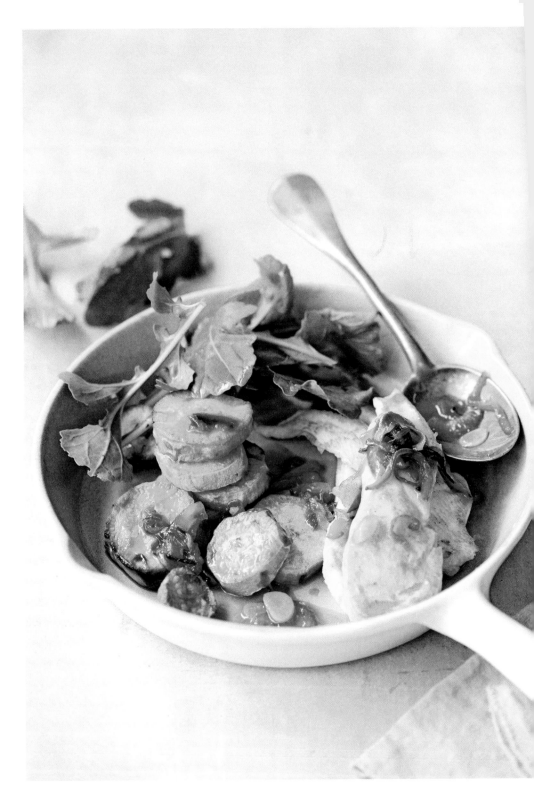

THE
NORDIC
WAY

*Discover the World's Most Perfect
Carb-to-Protein Ratio for
Preventing Weight Gain or Regain, and
Lowering Your Risk of Disease*

ARNE ASTRUP,
JENNIE BRAND-MILLER,
AND CHRISTIAN BITZ

PAM KRAUSS BOOKS / AVERY
NEW YORK

an imprint of Penguin Random House LLC
375 Hudson Street
New York, New York 10014

Most Avery books are available at special quantity discounts for bulk purchase for sales promotions, premiums, fund-raising, and educational needs. Special books or book excerpts also can be created to fit specific needs. For details, write SpecialMarkets@penguinrandomhouse.com.

Library of Congress Cataloging-in-Publication Data

Names: Astrup, Arne (Arne Vernon), author. | Brand Miller, Janette, 1952-
    author. | Bitz , Christian, author.
Title: The Nordic way / Arne Astrup, Jennie Brand-Miller, and Christian Bitz.
Description: New York : Pam Krauss Books/Avery, 2017.
Identifiers: LCCN 2016058140 | ISBN 9780451495846 (hardback)
Subjects: LCSH: Diet—Scandinavia. | Cooking, Scandinavian. | Health. |
    BISAC: COOKING / Health & Healing / Low Carbohydrate. | COOKING / Regional
    & Ethnic / Scandinavian. | LCGFT: Cookbooks.
Classification: LCC RA784 .A88 2017 | DDC 641.5948—dc23
LC record available at https://lccn.loc.gov/2016058140
p.   cm.

ISBN 9780451495846

Printed in the United States of America
10 9 8 7 6 5 4 3 2 1

Book design by Jan Derevjanik

Contents

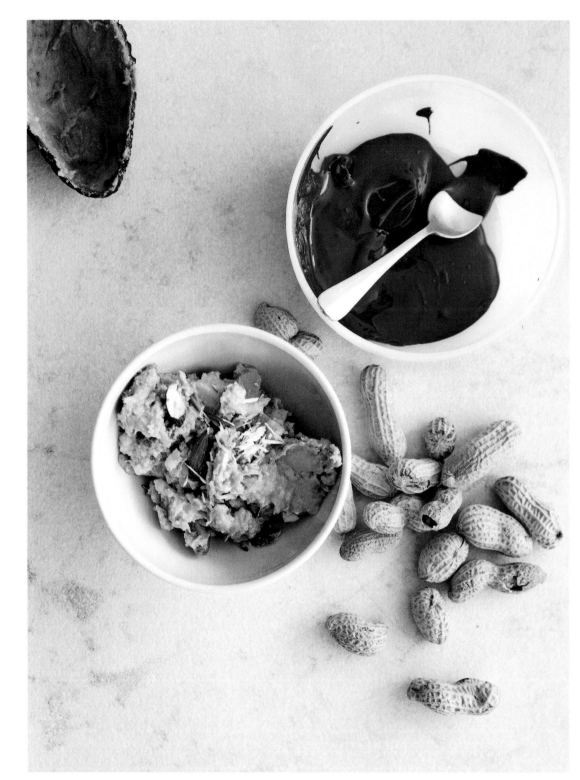

It's *Not* a Diet!

IN MAY 2016, THE *NEW YORK TIMES* PUBLISHED A FRONT-PAGE STORY CONFIRM-
ing a discouraging truism that millions of dieters recognized all too well: While
losing weight is hard, keeping it off is harder. So hard, in fact, that even dieters who had successfully shed a hundred pounds or more—sometimes much
more—were unable to keep off the weight they'd lost without enduring punish-
ing deprivation that was simply unsustainable. Small wonder that many readers
interpreted these findings as proof that sustained weight loss is simply unachiev-
able, and that to the contrary, our bodies are hard-wired to want to gain weight,
whether slowly, as a consequence of aging, or more rapidly, as a response to
severe calorie restriction.

Every day millions of Americans are engaged in what can feel like a losing
battle to maintain a normal weight and avoid the debilitating lifestyle conditions and diseases that can result from a typical Western convenience diet. You
may be one of them. If so, this meal plan (let's not call it a diet, even though it
will help you lose a few pounds) is for you. Perhaps you are looking to control
your blood pressure before resorting to medication. Maybe you're concerned
about the effects of inflammation. You may even have been alerted by your
doctor that you have prediabetes, and are at risk of developing type 2 diabetes
unless you lose weight. Or maybe you just want to improve your quality of life
by feeling fitter, leaner, and less encumbered. If any of these apply to you, you'll
find eating as the Scandinavian people traditionally have—a diet science now

recognizes as the very healthiest you can eat—will help you achieve your goals, and it will get you there without restricting or even counting calories. Nor will you need to eliminate entire categories of food from your life. That's because the Nordic Way is not a diet, but rather an old-is-new approach to eating that will support longevity and health; result in slow, sustainable weight loss; and prevent age-related weight creep.

Eating the Nordic Way—the way most Scandinavian people have eaten for generations, with an emphasis on nutritionally dense foods like unprocessed whole grains, high-fiber vegetables like cabbage, omega-rich fatty fish, and protein-packed dairy products—will automatically deliver these benefits, including an almost effortless approach to getting your weight under control. By now you've probably realized that losing weight isn't the problem—virtually any of the extreme plans currently making the rounds will help you drop a few pounds in the short run. Keeping it off is the real challenge. If you are one of the many who started a diet with high hopes, only to lose some weight and then regain it all (and maybe even put on a bit more), you may have convinced yourself that lasting weight loss just isn't possible. But we three, trained scientists and nutritional experts all, *know* that it is. And here's why.

With the world's largest dietary study, "DiOGenes," funded by the European Commission (their equivalent of the NIH) with around $20 million, we finally have a breakthrough in understanding how and why the diet is so crucial for optimal health, and particularly how you can maintain a healthy body weight and reduce inflammation in the body and diabetes risk without even *thinking* about calories . . . This important new research is the foundation of the principles in this book, and the findings are so compelling that we don't consider it hyperbole to call *The Nordic Way* the *most* effective meal plan for taming inflammation in the body and preventing weight gain for a lifetime.

The beauty of the DiOGenes concept is that we are not going to tell you to count calories and consume fewer of them—after all, you have tried that, and that approach only works as long as you are motivated to stick to it. What we *are* going to teach you is how you can lose weight *without* counting calories, and in particular how to prevent weight regain while achieving myriad other health and well-being benefits. Best of all, it will also help forestall the gradual weight gain or "creep" we've come to regard as a normal part of aging. That might sound impossible, so ingrained has the inevitability of the so-called "middle age spread" become, but by following the simple guidelines in *The Nordic Way*, you'll learn it's surprisingly easy to hold those unwanted pounds at bay. In short, we promise you a simple approach to composing meals that allows you to enjoy eating without thinking about calories—all with scientifically documented effects on weight and health.

Moreover, *The Nordic Way* is based on ordinary food—the kind you can find in regular supermarkets and are already accustomed to eating with just a few tweaks. We'll woo you with dishes that are bursting with so much flavor, the whole family will happily join in. And we promise that once you get started, you will not want to stray from your new, healthier food habits, which will soon become second nature—and virtually invisible to the world at large. Our approach, derived from the results of the world's largest diet study, is based on combining a moderately high intake of protein with low-glycemic-index carbs in a specific ratio, so counting calories is not necessary. We will explain exactly how easy that is for family meals in the following chapters. All you have to do is eat and enjoy the right balance of tasty foods that make you and your whole family healthier while warding off unwanted weight gain—or regain.

To get started all you have to do is be ready to eat good food! We describe the simple principles that *The Nordic Way* involves, and have developed delicious recipes that you can follow in conjunction with our meal plans while you get started. After that, you can use our recipes and guidelines for choosing and combining healthy ingredients to supplement your family's favorite meals. We've seen thousands successfully make these small adjustments a permanent lifestyle change—and we are confident you will enjoy the same results.

Moreover, following these guidelines will never feel like a sacrifice; to the contrary, the Scandinavian cuisine that forms the cornerstone of our program is at once time-tested and cutting edge. The food world had recently embraced our foodways for its purity of flavor and elegant simplicity; it's not a coincidence that Noma restaurant in Copenhagen has been ranked the world's best restaurant four times.

With such delicious and simple international cuisine to inspire you and the promise that you never need to gain another pound, we feel certain you'll soon believe, as we do, that *The Nordic Way* is the *only* way to eat . . . for life.

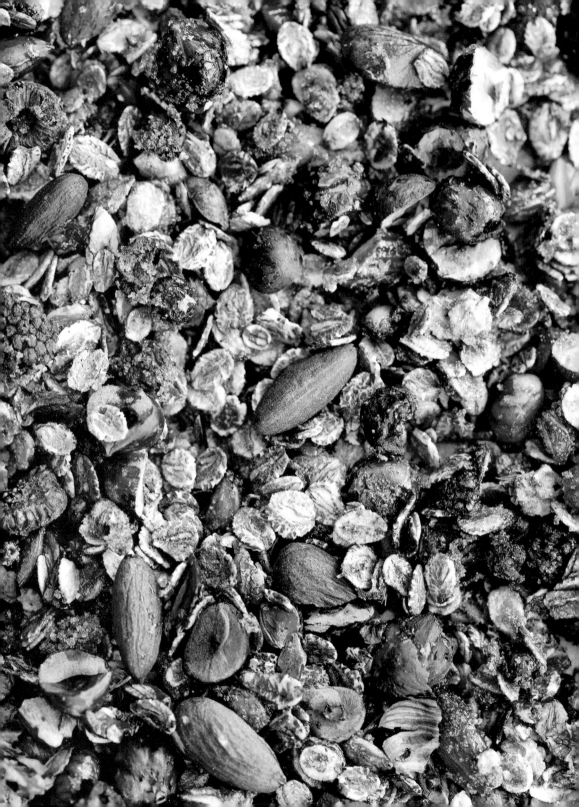

PART 1

THE SCIENCE BEHIND THE NORDIC WAY

THE NORDIC WAY IS ROOTED IN HISTORY AND THE TRADITIONAL FOODS COMMON to many populations throughout Scandinavia, but it took not one, not two, but three individuals trained in the science of food, nutrition, and physiology to connect the dots between those time-honored foodways, the latest breakthroughs in weight control, and a compellingly simple meal plan that is both appealing and effective in controlling weight. Surprisingly, though, this collaboration arose from conflict rather than a coming together of like-minded researchers.

In fact, it was more like brokering a peace treaty at the start! To provide a bit of background, Jennie is a leading scientist behind much of the groundbreaking research on the importance of the glycemic index (GI) of foods for stabilizing your blood glucose and promoting weight control and well-being. She has published many professional papers on the topic, as well as a number of books that have been bestsellers around the world. Arne, on the other hand, was a vocal opponent of the GI concept and considered the glycemic index too complex for non-academics or medical professionals to apply to their daily diets and, even more important, did not believe in the efficacy of lowering GI as a way to promote weight loss. After his research group in Copenhagen conducted a small study that essentially found lowering the overall GI of an individual's diet for a period of ten weeks did not really reduce body weight or body fat, Arne published the study in the *American Journal of Clinical Nutrition*, taking the debate public on an international scale. Jennie wrote a rather pointed "Letter to the Editor" criticizing the study as too small in scope, observing too few overweight subjects to have statistical significance. Her letter was published in the journal, and as a result, scientists all around the globe who studied obesity divided into two camps: those who saw the glycemic index as an important tool in the fight to control weight, and those who discounted it as useless.

In order to settle the dispute once and for all, Arne resolved to undertake the largest GI trial ever. Funded by more than $20 million from the European Commission research program, the study would observe overweight adults and children for more than six months, allowing Arne's team to accumulate data with sufficient statistical power to support his "no effect" conclusion. The large-scale study, dubbed DiOGenes (short for Diet and Obesity Genes) would be conducted in eight European research centers and reflect the results of more than a thousand participants, both adults and children.

Over the course of five years, more than forty-five scientists worked day and night on the study, and it was an exciting day when the statistician announced they were ready to release their findings. Much to Arne's astonishment, his theory was not supported by the research. To the contrary: it showed indisputably that even a small reduction in the GI of some key dietary items, in combination with a modest increase in protein intake, is sufficient to completely block weight gain. With such compelling evidence of its efficacy, Arne felt it was time to recognize the glycemic index concept as a valuable tool to control body weight.

With the study's publication in the *New England Journal of Medicine*, Arne announced his change of heart to the world—and two former opponents agreed to bury the hatchet. In fact, so profound was Arne's turnaround on the power of the glycemic index as a tool in the fight against weight gain that he and Jennie agreed to join forces in an effort to spread the message about the GI concept, Arne from Copenhagen, and Jennie from her home in Sydney, Australia.

All this new data was deeply encouraging, promising to offer consumers a scientifically sound road map to a healthier, trimmer life. But how to bridge the gap between the lab and the kitchen table? In order for these dietary guidelines to be effective outside of a clinical setting, they would need to be translated into a meal plan that was both simple to follow and flexible enough to live with indefinitely. Furthermore, the food on this plan should be so delicious that even those unwilling to sacrifice the very real pleasures of eating might be inspired to make a permanent lifestyle change in the name of health. No small order.

Enter the third leg of our stool, Christian Bitz. At that time, Christian was a very promising student of human nutrition in the University of Copenhagen's Department of Nutrition, Exercise and Sports, the largest institution of its kind in Europe. Arne, who is a professor and head of this department, was Christian's master thesis supervisor. Rather than pursue a PhD, however, Christian opted to pursue a career in TV, and is now one of the leading health communicators in Denmark. He also became the research director in clinical nutrition at two major hospitals in Copenhagen. Together, Christian and Arne wrote about the DiOGenes study and meal plans in Danish, and the resulting book—much of it the basis of the book you are now reading—went on to become a bestseller in Denmark, selling more than 250,000 copies in a country with a population of only 5.5 million people. Since then, Christian and Arne have worked closely together, combining their work with Jennie's to show that it is restriction of high GI carbohydrates, not calories, that is the key to achieving and maintaining weight loss. The result is a brand-new way of losing weight and, just as important, maintaining your current weight, whether you're coming off a significant weight loss or just hoping to stave off those gradual but insidious gains of a pound here and there that seem to sneak up on us all.

Because this book is all about preventing incremental weight gain or "creep" (the kind that adds up year after year) and preventing regain after weight loss, you'll get the best results if you are within a few pounds of your optimal weight when you begin. *The Nordic Way* is not designed to promote rapid weight loss (see page 15 for protocols we have found most effective for jump-starting your weight stabilization goals). Once you are where you want to be—or if you are there already—our program will help you stay there without feeling like your life is one perpetual diet. At the same time, you'll gain a host of health benefits that optimize your metabolism, preventing inflammation and cutting the risk that you'll develop type 2 diabetes, heart disease, of suffer from dementia or cancer as you grow older.

THE WORLD'S LARGEST DIETARY STUDY

Denmark is a small country (again, only 5.5 million people) and the capital city of Copenhagen is just one third the size of New York City, but Copenhagen University is one of the world's leading centers for nutrition research and the epicenter of Arne's study of the effect of foods, meals, and drinks on health and weight control.

The DiOGenes study is the largest of its kind and has been carried out in eight European countries with a total budget of more than $20 million including support from the European Union. The first and most important results were announced in November 2010 in the world's finest medical journal, *New England Journal of Medicine*, as well as in *Circulation* and *Pediatrics*.

The aim of the DiOGenes study was to compare the official dietary recommendations in Europe, which are very similar to American ones, with a diet based on the newest nutrition knowledge in a large group of European families, totaling 938 overweight adult family members and 827 children.

THE DIOGENES STUDY

We tested four new dietary patterns with different amounts of protein and types of carbohydrates against conventional national recommendations to find the one pattern that worked best. We already knew that protein produces higher satiety than carbohydrates and fat, mainly due to a more powerful effect of protein on the satiety hormones GLP-1 and PYY, both released from the lower small intestine when protein and, to some extent, fat fragments enter. Two diets had high protein and two had average levels, and two had low-glycemic-index carbs and two had high. The term *glycemic index* (GI) is one you may already be familiar with—it's used for classifying the impact of carbohydrates on the blood glucose (or blood sugar). If a food has a low GI, it means that it increases your blood glucose more slowly after consumption compared with a high-GI food.

It should be noted that the adults in the study came to it having been on a regimen of meal replacements for eight weeks to lose at least 8 percent of their weight before we started our phase of the investigation. This is because the *focus* of the study was to work out *how to keep weight off after it had been lost*. However, we have subsequently come to appreciate that this plan can be used as a weight loss program in its own right, resulting in a gradual loss of 2 to 4 pounds per week, as well as a highly effective hedge against the incremental weight gain that is associated with aging.

After losing weight, the participants were randomly divided into five different diet types (see box, page 16). In total, 548 participants completed the six-month dietary intervention. The results were striking: 30 percent fewer participants of the high-protein/low-GI group gave up halfway through the project compared with the group prescribed a lower-protein/high-GI diet. The group who ate high-protein/low-GI foods also performed best—and actually lost another half kilo *without trying* over the next six months rather than gaining! The remarkable thing was that in spite of the fact that they had just lost 20 pounds, the high-protein/low-GI dietary recommendations were able to keep them satisfied and full. Contrast that with the group assigned to the standard dietary recommendations—they gained back 5 pounds and many more gave up because of this!

Fortunately, we were able to keep following our participants because it was exciting to see that, over time, the results got better and better. The dieters in the high-protein/low-GI group continued to keep their weight off, and by the twelve-month mark were down more than 10 pounds compared to the group who used the national dietary recommendations. Results this clean-cut are rare in science and demonstrate that the key to keeping weight off is a diet rich in protein, with more lean meat and dairy products, lentils and beans, and fewer high-GI grains and grain-based products. You can eat until you are full without counting calories and enjoy what you are eating. Doesn't that sound good?

Over time, results from the DiOGenes study have continued to illustrate how important this dietary profile is—not just for adults but also for children. In the families where parents were assigned to the high-protein/low-GI diet group, the proportion of overweight children dropped markedly. There was no need to put the children on a diet or restrict their food. Just by eating with their parents according to the Nordic Way principles, they slimmed down without any direct intervention.

Many scientific studies have shown that people who are prone to gain weight find it easy to overeat even while following official dietary recommendations. Our goal with *The Nordic Way* was to construct a way of eating that is so filling that overeating isn't automatic—in other words, you don't have to count calories to stay slim and you don't have to stop eating until you are full.

WHY THIS IS NEWS

Over the past thirty years, consumers have been bombarded with diet books, many making extravagant claims and utilizing questionable methods, each and every one of which promised that their particular solution would unlock the secret to permanent weight loss. Of course, if even one of them had truly delivered on that promise, there would have been no need for the next one. And yet they continue to flood the bookshelves and the airwaves.

Many diet books make it sound simple: Fasting for two days and then eating normally for five days, shunning some carbs or all carbs or most fats—or binging on "good" fats; all these and many other more or less creative concepts. And though many of these regimens are harshly restrictive and in some cases less than palatable, many of the principles behind them are indeed scientifically proven to promote weight loss—in the short term. No doubt they would probably also work in the longer term—if one could stick to the meal plans. The fact is, if you eliminate and ban multiple foods and drinks from your diet, it is actually difficult to *avoid* losing weight, particularly if you eliminate all carbs. But saying good-bye permanently to so many foods you love is not sustainable in the long term. Few of us have the willpower to resist eating bread, rice, pasta, or cheese forever.

However, there is a nugget of truth in some of these books. Take, for example, the classic low-fat diet. There is no question that you will lose a few pounds if you shift from a high-fat diet to one lower in fats, but if you want to lose 10, 20, or 30 pounds, you will probably be disappointed—especially once you find that a number of your favorite foods are prohibited entirely. The same applies to the Atkins diet and the other extremely low-carbohydrate diets. These meal plans, which double your protein intake, are actually quite effective in making you feel full, so you do lose weight, particularly if you are insulin resistant or perhaps even prediabetic. (If insulin has a weak effect in your body, your disposal of sugar in the blood into the cells is compromised, and you will not obtain the satiety and fullness that are required to automatically stop your eating when you have consumed the calories your metabolism requires. But your blood sugar excursions will also be more pronounced, and increase the risk of diabetes and increase inflammation in the body.) But virtually all scientific investigations of these very-low-carbohydrate diets show that they cannot be sustained over time, and after a while, more or less all the weight that was shed is gained back. Most of us simply can't give up whole food groups like carbs on a permanent basis. It's a struggle to cross carbohydrates such as pasta, rice, potatoes, couscous, bulgur, oatmeal, muesli, cornflakes, fruit, berries, honey, and sugar off the menu for good. The same holds true for an extremely low-fat diet, which prohibits a lot of delicious foods that contain small amounts of fat. Who would want to commit to saying "no thanks" to a juicy steak, avocado, or cheese for the rest of their life?

The Nordic Way proposes a different approach. We don't ban *any* food group, and we encourage you to really enjoy your food by satisfying all five tastes (sweet, sour, salty, bitter, and umani). In fact, the participants in our studies were much less likely to opt out when their meal plans provided both enjoyment and satiety.

Our research and that of other nutrition scientists has shown that the body's food regulation mechanisms are complicated, but that one thing is quite simple: in order to sustainably control our weight over periods of months and years, we have to be able to both stay satisfied *and* enjoy food—preferably three times a day! A food culture in which whole food groups are left out is simply too restrictive for enjoyment and long-term sustainability. Still, we can learn something from these diets—for example, that too much fat in the food makes it easy to overeat and so causes weight gain. And so do refined grains and products made from them, such as soft white bread and fluffy rice. A little more protein is good for us, but extreme advice on protein or fat or carbs makes weight control harder rather than easier. The happy conclusion here is that moderation actually works best, which is why *The Nordic Way*, with its delicious meal plans, has been proven to help prevent weight gain—without discipline and deprivation.

It is also uniquely effective in preventing weight *re*gain after a more re-strictive diet, refuting assertions by some researchers that an inherited slow metabolism is the inevitable physiological response to extreme weight loss. We discovered some diet compositions enhance satiety, reduce hunger, and increase

GLYCEMIC INDEX

The glycemic index (GI) of a food is a number from 0 to 100 that is measured in the laboratory as the average increase of the blood glucose in the two hours after consumption compared with a reference food containing the same amount of carbohydrate. That may sound like a strangely specific measurement, but in fact all GI studies all over the world follow this exact protocol so the values are directly comparable. Nowadays, all GI values are defined relative to glucose (sometimes called dextrose), which has a GI of 100. Foods with a high GI (70 or above), such as white bread, rice, most varieties of potatoes, and jelly beans, will quickly raise blood glucose to a high level. Foods with a low GI (55 and below), such as some whole-grain breads, beans, pasta, dairy foods, and most fruit are broken down and absorbed more slowly, which causes a lower and more manageable increase in blood glucose.

Over the last fifteen years, researchers from all over the world have had a heated debate on whether GI can also be an effective tool in the fight against the excess weight. Indeed, apart from Jennie, we were against the concept initially because the scientific evidence was inconsistent. The results of the DiOGenes study convinced us that Jennie was right and that GI should be embraced.

There is a range of factors that influence the GI of a food—for example, particle size, fat, protein, and acid content. Because of this, GI cannot be used in isolation to determine whether a food is healthy or not. As an example, potato chips made from potatoes fried in large amounts of fat have a lower GI than boiled white potatoes. The reason for this is that fat lowers the absorption rate of carbohydrates and so the GI is lowered. For this reason, many cakes and biscuits will have a low GI because they are full of fat. See the chart on page 37 for more factors that have an influence on the GI of a meal. But no matter what, you will lose weight more easily and achieve significant health benefits if you replace the high-GI foods in your diet with their low-GI counterparts.

metabolism better than others, and thereby enable people to stop eating after having consumed the number of calories they need to keep the reduced body weight stable.

The DiOGenes study showed that obese subjects who have lost 24 pounds over eight weeks on a calorie-restricted diet subsequently started to regain weight if they followed dietary guidelines that prescribed modest amounts of fat and protein together with more carbohydrate-rich foods. By contrast, those assigned a diet with slightly reduced carbohydrate intake chosen from a selection of low-GI foods did not regain *any* body weight over six months—despite their being allowed to eat freely until they felt full and satiated.

CARBS VS. PROTEIN: THE GOLDEN RATIO

In *The Nordic Way*, our recommended ratio of carbs to protein is 2:1 (and we will explain exactly how we arrived at that formula in a bit). In round numbers, that means eating about 200 grams of carbohydrates and 100 grams of protein per day. But an important question is whether you should consider eating even fewer carbs, or skip them altogether. There is no doubt that low-carb diets (those that restrict carbohydrate intake to about 50 grams a day) are very effective for weight loss, and also to prevent and treat type 2 diabetes. You might have tried one of them and experienced the effects on your own body. They are most effective in individuals with a poor insulin action, such as those with prediabetes, type 2 diabetes, polycystic ovarian syndrome (PCOS), or psoriasis, and less effective among the more physically active and those with a genetically determined good insulin sensitivity.

On a severely carb-restricted diet, while you'll be able to eat more good fats and protein from healthy sources (nuts, avocados, fatty fish, etc.) and more salad and vegetables, many of your favorite foods are off the menu. Most such diets require you to *severely* restrict grains and grain-based foods (bread, pasta, rice), starchy vegetables (potatoes), most types of fruit (apples, bananas), chocolate, and desserts. In the short term—say two to three months of active weight loss—that's tolerable, but what about for the rest of your life, when *maintaining* your new weight is the goal?

Studies show that while it is possible to completely skip all the carbohydrates you love for some weeks or even a few months, most people cannot go on the rest of their lives without bread, pasta, rice, couscous, fruit, berries, etc. A low-carb diet makes life tough, requiring a lot of discipline and self-sacrifice, and the chances that you will go off the rails is high. Your family and friends won't be thrilled, either. And they may well ask if your eating plan is good for the planet. On top of all that, as soon as you start eating carbs again, you will regain the weight you have lost. In *The Nordic Way*, we base our recommendations on the basis of studies in both science and humanities. The social and environmental consequences of our eating patterns must be considered, too.

For this reason, we recommend a *modestly* higher-protein, lower-carbohydrate diet for longer-term weight control and gradual, truly sustainable weight loss. You are allowed to eat your carbs in just *slightly* lower amounts than what you're used to, and they can remain on your plate because the lower GI carbs do not have the same adverse effect on your health. Indeed, it is better to eat low-GI carbs than to skip them because they reduce inflammation in your body, and when you are still allowed to eat your beloved carbs, you can better stick to the meal plan than if they were banned.

SATIETY IS THE WAY TO BECOME SLIM

The traditional advice the American population has received to reduce weight and maintain a healthy body weight is to restrict the amount of consumed calories—"Eat less." This approach has proven very ineffective, and the reason is quite obvious: Nobody has given more specific advice about how to suppress the driver of the excessive calorie intake—namely hunger and lack of real satiety. Conversely, when you eat foods and meals that provide you with more satiety and fullness, you will automatically, without really thinking about it, consume fewer calories.

Over the past twenty-five years, Jennie and Arne have been working independently to discover how to create greater satiety with fewer calories and without eliminating entire food groups. "Satiety," by the way, is the scientific name for that elusive, wonderful sensation of fullness at the end of the meal that tells us we have had enough. If we can both eliminate constant hunger pangs *and* create enjoyable satiety, we have the best defense against overeating at meals and snack times.

In other words, the solution to long-term successful weight control is feeling sufficiently full and satisfied at the end of eating, so hunger takes hours to return.

Unfortunately, this is not as simple as stuffing yourself with low-calorie foods. If you subsist on cabbage soup, there is no doubt that you will lose weight, but you will have compromised on taste and the food culture you live in to an intolerable degree. We need our senses—not just our stomachs—to feel satisfied; food has to taste good and it has to allow you to take part in the social interactions we all cherish and that make life worthwhile.

APPETITE VERSUS HUNGER

There is a difference between appetite and hunger. Hunger is a biological drive—a survival mechanism that is regulated by how much food we eat and have in our stomach. Hunger is thus entirely controlled by inner physiological mechanisms. Appetite, on the other hand, is a psychological desire for specific food, which is regulated by factors such as habits and the scent and sight of food. You can be hungry and have no appetite or desire to eat, for example, when you are sick. Conversely, you can have an appetite and not be hungry, for example, at the sight of a delicious dessert after a main course. This is the reason that satiety is not the opposite of being hungry. Satiety is stimulated in a different area of the brain from hunger and, unlike hunger, is also affected by our appetite. In order to experience a satisfying feeling of satiety, both appetite and hunger need to be addressed! A meal of low-fat vegetables is unsatisfying even if it is filling, and why *The Nordic Way* is based on food that is satisfying as well as hunger-reducing.

FEEDING BODY AND SOUL
THE HYGGE WAY

In Scandinavia, we have a term called *hygge* that can be hard to pronounce and even harder to explain. *Hygge* (pronounced *hyooga*) translates roughly as cozy, homey, informal, sincere, down-to-earth, warm, close, convivial, relaxed, comfortable, snug, friendly, welcoming, and tranquil. It is a notion that is central to our home life and also applies to how we think about food, eating, and entertaining.

Hygge's etymological origin lies in the Norwegian language (and, further back, Old Norse), and references to its meaning in eighteenth-century Norwegian center on such things as the safe habitat; the experience of comfort and joy, especially in one's home and family; a caring orientation, for example, toward children; a civilized mode of behavior that other people find easy to get along with, one that soothes them and builds their trust; a house that, while not splendid or overly stylish, is respectably clean and well kept.

Hygge signifies a safe, low-key, intimate form of socialization. For many people, the notion of having "a *hyggelig* time" is being with good friends or with one's family or partner, having fun in an easy-going, not overly stimulating way. The home seems to be the most common setting for *hygge*, although social encounters in other locations can also easily be seen as *hyggelig*. People experience a sense of closeness, often based on sharing food and drinks (with or without alcohol).

When we designed the food component of *The Nordic Way*, we were very mindful of the traditions around food and conviviality that the Scandinavian people hold dear, and for that reason, ours may be the only eating plan that can be said to be both scientifically proven *and hyggelig*. The food is comforting, familiar, soul-satisfying, and nourishing to both body and spirit. It is in deep contrast to most programs that focus on deprivation and what is eliminated. *The Nordic Way* is about embracing wholesome, satisfying ingredients in the proper balance, enjoying good food, and spending time with friends and family—a prescription anyone can follow with pleasure.

PALATABILITY
IS THE ROAD
TO SATISFACTION

We have deliberately designed *The Nordic Way* so that you can enjoy meals with family and friends. Moreover, it tastes so good that you will learn to *love* eating healthy food. In fact, we'd wager that you'll begin to wonder how you ever found the typical American diet palatable. This is not just because we want you to enjoy your food (though of course we do), but because our research shows that this is what works best—the less restrictive a dietary change is, and the fewer prohibitions of common foods it involves, the easier it is to stick to. The "science of weight control" turns out to *require* enjoyment, which is great news for people who have refused to eat healthy because they think it's all salads and seeds.

The British scientist Dr. Áine McConnon from the University of Surrey in the United Kingdom, who was a member of the scientific European DiOGenes consortium, analyzed the acceptability of the most successful DiOGenes food regimen that was used during the trial. In hindsight it is hardly surprising that the meal plans that were more enjoyable, easy, convenient, and satisfying than the others produced the best results! And these findings partially explain why so few study participants gave up and dropped out from the trial if they were in that diet group. Clearly palatability and enjoyment of the food are essential to long-lasting success, the kind so many of our study subjects were able to achieve.

THE FLAVOR FACTOR

A basic scientific principle of taste enjoyment that we use in *The Nordic Way* is to stimulate all our routes of sensory perception—taste, smell, touch, and the trigeminal sense triggered when the tongue is irritated by spicy food, for example (more about this in a minute), all of which are crucial for a pleasurable overall food experience.

The sense of taste can basically be divided into four basic tastes—sour, sweet, salty, and bitter—and a fifth taste, umami. All parts of the tongue can detect all tastes, but the grouping of taste cells is not the same throughout the tongue. The density of the different taste cells is divided as follows: Sweet is mainly tasted on the front of the tongue, bitter on the back, and sour and salty along the sides. Salt sensitivity is mainly tasted in the front. Umami is also called the third spice. The taste of umami is complicated to define, but is described by some as a meaty quality. It is mainly tasted on the back of the tongue and adds more flavor to the food.

The sense of smell is particularly important for the flavor of food. Just think about how the food tastes, or precisely how it does not taste, when your nose is blocked when you have a cold. The nose has more than one thousand olfactory receptors, which make the sense of smell far more nuanced than the sense of taste. The sense of smell is engaged before the food is eaten, but it also comes into play while you are chewing your food, because flavors are released that reach the receptors in the nose through the throat. The odor signals are integrated with other senses inside the brain itself, and this integration gives the complete sensory experience. The sense of smell can also be overstimulated so it actually curbs the appetite. A good example of this is if you have spent several hours preparing food for guests and then find you have no appetite once you finally get seated.

The sense of touch is often related to the texture and structure of the foods in the context of "mouthfeel." Textural contrasts between crispy and soft, for example, contribute to optimal satisfaction—just think about the texture of a macaron, the crispness of the shell and the chewy, soft center; or the way a KitKat "cracks" and then melts in the mouth. We can also make use of this in the healthy cuisine where, for example, sprinkling roasted sliced almonds onto a salad adds a nice crunchy contrast to the softer vegetables.

The sense of sight is also important for our choice of food. Just think about a tempting ice cream sign on a hot summer day. It is primarily based on associations connected with taste and thus is not a part of the direct sensation in the mouth. But the sight can have great importance for our desire to eat—or the lack thereof.

In addition to these four senses, there is the essential fifth sense: the trigeminal sense. This sense is stimulated by "irritations" of the tongue, the throat, or the inside of the nose. The burning sensation of hot peppers, mustard, and ginger and the fizzing of champagne are examples of trigeminal stimulation.

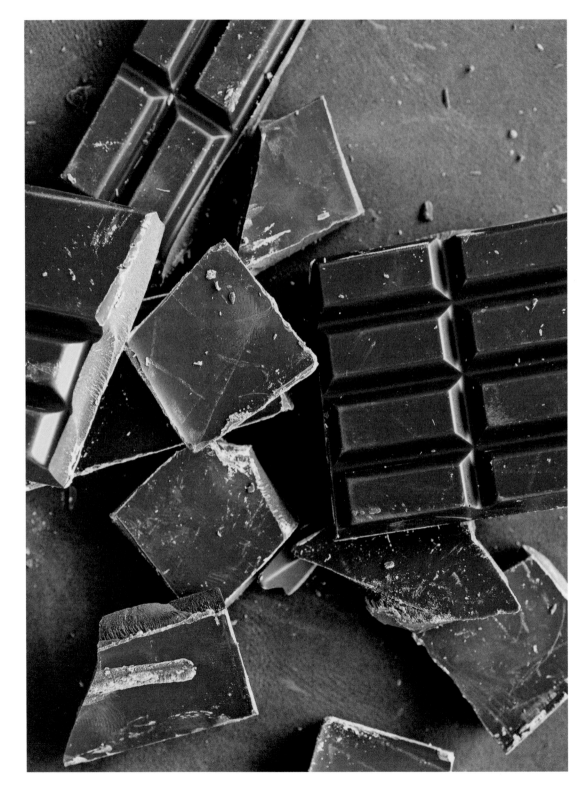

There is now solid evidence that our appetite is satisfied faster if the food "tastes like something" and hits all the five taste senses.

Cooking to engage all these senses might seem like a complicated affair, but that doesn't have to be the case. Start by thinking in terms of foods with the five basic tastes as the key to a tasty and satisfying meal. A sandwich made on whole wheat bread (bitter) topped with roasted chicken (umami and salt) and pickles (sour/sweet) is an excellent example of this. The same applies to a pizza: ham or pepperoni (umami and salt), tomato sauce (sweet), and topped with fresh arugula (bitter)—and here we also get the contrast between the crispy bread and the soft cheese. But you do not have to have all five taste nuances in the same dish. You could serve a refreshing salad of bitter lettuces with a sweet-and-sour dressing with a main dish of meat or fish and plenty of vegetables. Round off the meal with a piece of good-quality dark chocolate, and you have a meal that satisfies all five taste senses! Dividing the meal into several dishes moreover has the advantage of helping you to eat more slowly, which also improves satiety.

INDULGENCE

We, as human beings, have a strong need for indulgence. Some scientists believe it is one of the strongest driving forces in our lives. Most of us find indulgence and reward in the food we eat—for example, a small dessert (Jennie says two squares of high-quality chocolate) after a hard day at work. Or a well-deserved beer on Friday after a long week. The important thing to know here is that it is quite easy to develop habits that feel indulgent but really are not in absolute terms. If we are told a sufficient number of times that a bowl of sweet ripe strawberries is the ultimate treat, in the end we believe it! We can use this mechanism to continue to feel indulged even while largely giving up all the very rich foods that caused us to gain weight.

While you are on the four-week *The Nordic Way* plan, you should "train" your sense of indulgence. What do you really appreciate? And can you get the same indulgence by eating it in smaller amounts, but with full attention? Can you perhaps replace some of your unhealthy habits with some that are a little healthier? It's a great habit to acquire, because it will have a big impact on your weight.

Remember, too, that you can sin with style! For sure, don't waste calories on junk that doesn't even taste good, but occasionally it is fine to go off the healthy path as long as you get back on it promptly. Research has shown that for many people, it is actually easier to keep a healthy lifestyle if you let yourself go once in a while. Not all the time, but, for example, on a Saturday night—and with good conscience. Feel how the strength is running through your body when you have only one glass of wine or eat only a modest slice of cake. Or maybe even say "no, thank you" to the second glass. It is important that you enjoy the indulgences you do have and also work on controlling temptation, so that you can enjoy with good conscience those times when you stray from the plan.

CAN YOU EAT TOO MUCH MEAT?

Scientific studies suggest that eating large amounts of processed red meat may increase the risk of cancer and heart disease. For that reason, *The Nordic Way* emphasizes other good protein sources including fish, poultry, legumes, and dairy products. It is also useful to know that not all red meats are equally harmful. For example, gentle cooking processes like boiling or slow roasting at low temperatures do not produce the high levels of carcinogens found in smoked, grilled, and browned foods, as well as industrially processed meats such as cold cuts with added salt, nitrites, and other undesirable ingredients.

HOW SLIM DO
YOU WANT TO BE?

After weight loss, you are usually on your own, but this is where *The Nordic Way* continues! We hope that you will find it a specific and simple diet to follow, and that you will develop a foundation of healthier habits that you do not want to abandon! All you have to do is follow the template of our suggested menus while you integrate the principles of the plan into your everyday life. Use those same principles to design your own meals that adhere to our 2:1 ratio overall. You cannot and should not be on a diet the rest of your life. And you do not need to.

You might have heard of the dieters who succeeded in losing large amounts of weight—the so-called biggest losers—but ultimately regained most if not all of their lost weight. Frankly, these findings were not surprising to us. Weight loss experts have been prescribing "cut down on calorie intake" for decades, both to the overweight public and as part of management programs for severely obese people. This approach does not work in the long term for the simple reason that the underlying cause of gain weight has not been neutralized, and will work with full power to force the caloric intake up again once the calorie-counting exercise stops. An important underlying cause is the composition of the diet. The relapse is not due to an inherited slow metabolism the obese people have to live with, as suggested by some studies. There is actually a way to prevent weight regain and normalize metabolism without hunger and calorie counting, and the DiOGenes study shows the way!

During our many years of working with overweight people, we have seen a lot of people who have been on a diet and lost weight. For most people, the challenge is keeping the weight down. But this is exactly what *The Nordic Way* is created for. Our diet composition is literally the best in the world for maintaining weight loss, as proven in the DiOGenes study. And the great thing is you can do this without feeling deprived.

In addition to your weight loss, you will probably notice the many positive health-related consequences of your new diet. But you will probably also experience that there are things that do not fit into a busy schedule or foods you have missed. This is okay, because it is important that you adjust the principles to fit you and your life and not the other way around.

Nothing is prohibited or wrong, as long as you are conscious of your choices and as long as you are prioritizing your health.

This eating plan enhances satiety, reduces hunger, and increases metabolism better than others, and thereby enables people to stop eating after having consumed the amount of calories they need to keep the reduced body weight stable.

There is growing evidence that the obesity epidemic has coincided with the dramatically increased consumption of refined carbohydrates such as bread, rice, and juice. Susceptible individuals respond with overconsumption of calories, resulting in weight gain. This has helped us to understand that the carbohydrates present in different foods have distinct physiological effects, including those on postprandial glycemia and insulinemia, which can influence the rate of digestion, appetite (hunger and satiety), fuel partitioning, and metabolic rate. The quality of carbohydrate is most relevant to individuals who are overweight and at increased risk of diabetes mellitus. The glycemic index (GI) is a food classification derived from the postprandial blood glucose response relative to a reference food, gram for gram of carbohydrate. The glycemic load (GL)—the mathematical product of the GI and the amount of carbohydrate—encapsulates both the quality and quantity of carbohydrate, and is the single best predictor of postprandial glycemia.

In overweight and insulin-resistant individuals consuming high-GI and/or -GL diets, glycemic spikes and insulin demand are excessively increased. Overweight and obese individuals following ad libitum low-GI or low-GL diets lose more fat mass than those on a conventional low-fat diet. In pioneering work, Professor David Ludwig from Boston has shown that compared with a conventional low-fat diet, following a low-GL diet produced markedly greater decreases in weight and body fat among obese adults with high levels of insulin secretion. The same group of scientists have pointed out that reduced energy expenditure following a period of weight loss can be normalized by following a low-GL or low-GI diet.

Taken together, the various studies outlined above demonstrate the importance of considering dietary composition in any weight-management program, and in particular for weight maintenance and prevention of relapse after a major weight loss.

SINCE THE DANISH EDITION OF *THE NORDIC WAY* (IN DANISH: *VERDENS BEDSTE Kur*) was published in Denmark, we have analyzed more results of the long-term effects. From the DiOGenes study, which is the strongest scientific documentation of the world's best diet, we now know that:

1. The food plan is so easy that the dropout rate over fourteen months was halved compared to those who ate a typical low-fat diet (normal protein content and a higher GI).

2. The weight loss difference between the Nordic Way program and other groups continued to increase—in fact, the difference doubled!

3. Comprehensive analyses of taste preferences carried out by British researchers, as a part of the DiOGenes study, show that the test subjects loved the food. It's not just the superior weight control our food plan provides; the high continuation rate of people in our study suggests the food also tastes better (a thesis you will be able to put to the test yourself with the recipes starting on page 69).

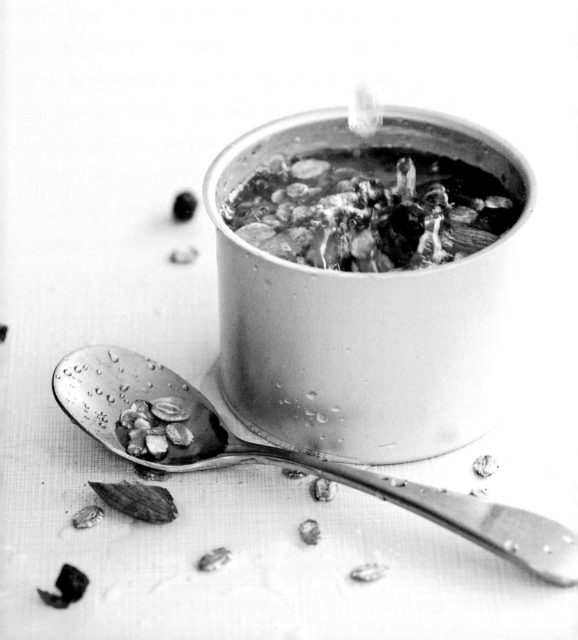

PART 2

MAKING THE NORDIC WAY PRINCIPLES WORK FOR YOU

BY NOW WE HOPE YOU HAVE A CLEAR UNDERSTANDING OF THE PRINCIPLES that govern the Nordic Way. But theory is one thing—practice is another. Once again, we do want to stress that this is *not* a diet meant to result in rapid weight loss over a short period of time. *This is a food manual for life.* This chapter gives you the specific tools for using the program every day, on an ongoing basis. We have developed lists and advice for you to use when you are grocery shopping, preparing food, and eating at home or in restaurants. We are convinced that you will become comfortable with the principles fast, so that eating and composing menus the Nordic Way will soon become habit.

WHAT TO PUT IN YOUR SHOPPING CART

The first step in shifting your eating and cooking habits to the Nordic Way is choosing foods with a low GI. If a food has a low GI, it means that it will cause your blood sugar to rise more slowly, and to a lower level, compared to foods with a high GI. Carbohydrate foods include all varieties of fruit, starchy vegetables like potatoes (not salad vegetables), dairy products like milk and yogurt (but not cheese), grains and grain products such as bread and pasta, and beans and legumes. Only foods containing carbohydrates can have a GI value.

Most fruits have a low GI and can therefore be eaten freely. Apples, pears, oranges, bananas, blueberries, and strawberries are all good to go. A small number of fruits, such as watermelon, have a high GI, but they happen to be the ones that don't contribute a lot of carbohydrate, so you *don't* need to restrict them. Nearly all vegetables have a low GI (even carrots!). The big exception is potatoes, which can still be eaten but not in large quantity. Carrots and beets have lots of color and contribute a big dose of antioxidants.

When it comes to grains and grain products, choose those proven to be low GI, preferably whole grains, which contain more micronutrients. Unfortunately, at this time, very few products are labeled low GI; in the United States, when in doubt, opt for kernel-heavy and dense breads made by traditional methods. Pumpernickel bread has the lowest GI of all commercially available breads (although it's not everyone's favorite!). A good alternative, if you can't make your own, is to buy genuine sourdough breads, those made with *authentic* sourdough starter by artisan bakers. These loaves have a low GI because the fermentation process produces lactic acid, which not only gives sourdough its unique taste but also slows down stomach emptying and prolongs the time your body needs to digest the food. When digestion takes longer, the food has less impact on blood sugar levels and helps you feel fuller longer.

Don't make the mistake of assuming that all whole-grain breads, especially soft and fluffy breads labeled "whole wheat," are low GI. In general, they have the same GI as white bread because they are made from flours that are finely milled, or from a mixture of whole and processed grains.

You may be surprised to learn that most varieties of pasta have a low GI, whether white or brown. Whole-grain pastas contain more nutrients, but if they are not to your taste, there's no need to "suffer" them (enjoying food takes precedence).

Most types of rice available in North America, whether white or brown, long grain or medium grain, have a moderate to high GI, but there are some important exceptions. Low-GI foods include basmati rice, Doongara rice, "converted" (parboiled) rice, and any type of quick-cooking rice that comes in a pouch. Sushi has a low GI for a variety of reasons, including the fact that it is eaten cold.

Choose breakfast cereals that are known to have a low GI (such as Kellogg's All-Bran or those containing a fiber called psyllium). If you are fond of hot oatmeal in winter, avoid the instant varieties (they have a *really* high GI) and instead go for steel-cut oats. They take a little longer to cook, but they are worth every minute.

Cooking starchy foods until well done and soft increases their GI, so always cook your pasta and rice al dente (until tender but still slightly chewy). Cooling also turns some starch into resistant starch that is more slowly digested, so a cold potato or rice salad has a lower GI than the same ingredients served hot.

Last but not least, be mindful of sugar. Of course, large amounts of sugar are not to be recommended, but there's no need to strictly avoid it. The World Health Organization recommends an individual derive no more than 10 percent of his energy (i.e., calories) in the form of free sugars, whether it's cane sugar, high-fructose corn syrup, maple syrup, brown rice syrup, or honey. For most people, that means you can consume about 50 grams a day, equivalent to about 12 teaspoons. This amount includes the added sugars found in processed foods like ketchup, and food labels will help you discover how much is lurking in the prepared foods you buy. That said, your allowance of free sugars is best used to increase your enjoyment of healthy foods such as whole-grain breads and rolls (a little jelly or marmalade on toast) or oat cereals (a little brown sugar or honey). Many yogurts on the market are highly sweetened, so we recommend that you mix them with an equal amount of unsweetened yogurt. That way you get a big serving of calcium, protein, and other nutrients without excessive sugar or calories.

In the chart on page 49, you will find a detailed list of foods and their GI values. More extensive lists of GI values can be found online (www.glycemicindex.com).

EXCHANGE YOUR HIGH, GI FAST CARBOHYDRATES FOR SLOW CARBOHYDRATES WITH A LOW GI

HI-GI FOODS	RECOMMENDED ALTERNATIVE
White bread (including bagels and burger buns)	Whole-grain bread, bread containing whole grains, or sourdough bread
Corn flakes, wheat flakes	An oat-based whole-grain breakfast cereal product (for example overnight oats) or products labelled "low GI"
Instant oatmeal	Steel-cut oatmeal
Rice, including long grain, Jasmine, Calrose	Basmati, low-GI varieties
Jelly beans, gummy bears	Nuts and dried fruit
Crackers	Unsweetened whole-grain oat biscuits

FACTORS INFLUENCING THE GI VALUES OF FOODS

FACTOR	MECHANISM	EXAMPLES
Starch "gelatinization"	When starchy foods are heated and/or put in water the starch swells, which increases the GI.	Pasta cooked al dente has a lower GI than when it is overcooked.
Processing	The fibrous shell of seeds, beans, and grains is a physical barrier against the breakdown and absorption of carbohydrates.	The more intact grains, seeds, and beans, etc., are the lower the GI.
Particle size	The finer the particle size the easier it is for water and enzymes to enter.	Finely ground flour has a higher GI than coarsely ground or stone-ground flour.
Sugar	Contrary to expectation, added sugar can actually contribute in lowering the GI of starchy products, as sugar among other things inhibits gelatinization.	Raisin breads and other sweet-tasting varieties have a lower GI than regular bread. Some sugar in/on breakfast cereals increases their palatability. However that sugar should be included in your daily allowance of 12 teaspoons.
Acid content	Tart, sour, and acidic foods make the stomach empty more slowly. This is a chemical effect on the ring of muscle called the pylorus. By reducing the rate of stomach emptying, the digestion of all carbohydrates in the intestine is also slowed. This is a good thing because that feeling of fullness—satiety—becomes more exaggerated. In the past, these foods were said to "stick to the ribs."	Vinegar, lemon juice, pickles, sourdough bread, etc., contribute to lowering the GI of a meal.
Fat	Fatty foods also send a signal to the pylorus to make the stomach empty more slowly. As a result, the absorption of all carbohydrates is slowed down and you feel fuller for longer.	Potato chips have a lower GI than boiled potatoes. If they are cooked in olive oil or other unsaturated fat, they are healthier. But beware—they are all too easy to overeat.
Types of starch	There are two types of starch, which are absorbed differently because of their structure, due to ease of gelatinization.	Basmati rice and some other varieties have lower GI than sticky rices such as jasmine (due to differences in type of starch).

HOW TO CHOOSE PROTEIN-RICH FOODS

In the Nordic Way program, protein makes up 20 to 30 percent of total calories consumed each day, which is optimal when it comes to preventing weight regain.

New research has shown that protein is better than carbohydrate at stimulating the release of satiety hormones like cholecystokinin (CCK). Receptors on the wall of the stomach detect the arrival of food and send a range of chemical signals (such as CCK) through the blood to the brain to indicate that digestion is taking place. Stomach emptying is slowed so that the small intestine receives food at a steady pace.

The most important satiety hormone, GLP-1, is secreted from cells in the lower part of the small intestine. Degradation fragments of protein and fats are particularly powerful signals to stimulate the release of GLP-1 from the small intestine into the bloodstream. So after you have eaten protein-rich meals, more GLP-1 will reach the brain and make you feel satiated.

All of which is a highly technical way of saying that consuming plenty of protein ensures you be satiated and thus will stop eating sooner. Foods such as lean meat, poultry, fish, eggs, and low-fat dairy products are all rich in protein and essential tools for hitting that desirable carb-to-protein ratio that is at the center of *The Nordic Way*'s approach to eating for lifelong health.

Examples of highly recommended proteins are shellfish, white and fatty fishes, skinless poultry, venison, lean pork, veal, lamb, and beef. Try to choose lean cuts with little or no marbling and remove any visible fat. You also need plenty of good low-fat dairy products—they are also rich in protein and contain calcium, which binds some of the fat. The low-fat dairy products used most often in our meal plans are nonfat and 1% milk, plain low-fat or fat-free Greek yogurt, and low-fat cottage cheese.

If you are a vegetarian or vegan, you can still choose a modestly higher-protein, lower-carbohydrate food plan. Tofu—a source of protein made from mashed soybeans—can feature prominently. Legumes in any shape or form are a great choice because they contain quite a lot of protein and their carbohydrate is low GI. Indeed, the ratio of carbohydrate to protein is perfect (about 2:1). Any recipe containing lentils, peas, or beans will be giving you the best of both worlds (higher protein *and* lower GI).

The chart on page 48 provides a detailed list of the most protein-rich foods to help you select the most satiating and slimming foods when you are grocery shopping.

WHAT ABOUT FIBER?

Many research studies show that dietary fiber—the parts of plants that are indigestible—are also good for satiety and are food for the microflora in your digestive system, or microbiome. We love fiber, too—it's an integral part of the *The Nordic Way* menus because the richest natural sources of fiber are vegetables and whole grains, which are a central part of the program. To increase the fiber content of your meals, sprinkle chia seeds on your foods. Chia is an excellent source of soluble, viscous fiber that not only slows down the digestion of all carbohydrates, but feeds your good microbes.

THE MAGIC RATIO:
FINDING YOUR BEST BALANCE
BETWEEN PROTEIN AND
CARBOHYDRATES

On our meal plans, you are likely to eat fewer carbohydrates and more protein than you have in the past. A typical American male eats 300 grams of carbohydrates and 100 grams of protein every day—this corresponds to a carbohydrates-to-protein ratio of about 3 to 1. The average American woman eats an even *more* carb-heavy diet: about 225 grams of carbohydrates and 68 grams of protein. On the whole, you should aim for your meal or recipe to have a ratio of carbs to protein of *2 or less*.

In practical terms, this means that every time you eat 50 grams of carbohydrates (including those from vegetables and fruits), it should be balanced by 25 grams of protein. Just as essential, most, if not all, of the carbs you *do* eat should be of the low-glycemic kind. Hitting this golden ratio of low-GI carbs to protein means you will be more satisfied, be less likely to overeat, and will maintain a healthy weight (or keep off any pounds you have recently shed) indefinitely. As in *forever*.

Every time you include a protein-rich food in a meal, it helps you to reach

---

IS THE RATIO OKAY?

10g carbohydrates and 2g protein = 10 / 2 = 5
(FAR TOO CARB-HEAVY)

10g carbohydrates and 5g protein = 10 / 5 = 2
(EXCELLENT–THE IDEAL RATIO)

10g carbohydrates and 10g protein = 10 / 10 = 1
(PROTEIN HEAVY, OKAY FOR OCCASIONAL MEALS)

10g carbohydrates and 15g protein = 10 / 15 = 0.66
(TOO PROTEIN HEAVY)

---

your protein target. Let's take yogurt as an example. The natural (unsweetened) low-fat varieties contain about 6 grams protein and 6 grams carbohydrate per 100 grams for a ratio of protein to carbs of 1:1. Perhaps you're thinking, *Hey, that's great! I'm actually doing* better *than the target goal if I take my yogurt plain.* But not only is eating plain, unsweetened yogurt not everyone's cup of tea, there's no reason not to make that yogurt as palatable and pleasant as possible on our plan. The point is not to eliminate any food group or to encourage you down the path of deprivation of protein-fueled eating. We want you to eat and enjoy carbohydrate-rich food—just of the right kind and in the right proportions. So to achieve the 2:1 ratio, you will need to add 6 grams of carbohydrates from another source, in this case, in the form of a little serving of fruit and/or honey with your yogurt. Just be sure that the total amount of carbs is never more than twice the protein.

Perhaps you are still thinking that a ratio of 1:1 (carbs to protein) might be better than 2:1? That might be okay for a lunch or dinner meal (e.g., steak, salad vegetables, and a small potato). But we recommend that you eat proportionately more carbs at breakfast so that the ratio for the whole day is 2:1. We say this because most people really enjoy carbohydrate foods, especially sweet ones. If you go without them entirely and feel deprived or unsatisfied by your overall diet, your natural urges might derail your whole diet. As we've noted in our research, a food pattern that requires a lot of self-sacrifice will not be one that sustains you all your life.

Here is a more specific example:

A good breakfast

Fruit (120 grams) and yogurt (200 grams)

The fruit contributes 12 grams carbohydrate but 0 gram protein.

The yogurt contributes 12 grams carbohydrate and 12 grams protein.

The carbohydrate content of the whole breakfast is: 12 grams + 12 grams = 24 grams.

The protein content in your breakfast: 0 + 12 grams = 12 grams.

So the ratio between carbohydrate and protein is 24:12—which means the ratio is 2:1.

If you need more calories (as a typical man probably would), you could eat proportionately more of both the fruit and the yogurt (say, 180 grams fruit and 300 grams yogurt). Alternately, you could add a few berries (for carbs) and a few nuts (for protein and fat) and have a delicious meal that perfectly fits the Nordic Way profile!

In terms of quantity, you should be guided by your natural appetite. Eat more if you want to, eat less if you prefer. Try to really *listen* to those signals inside your body. We have also inserted ratios for all the recipes in this book.

THE NORDIC WAY PLATE

When your meal is a traditional protein-carb-veggie plate, you can put together your meals on the basis of the plate model below:

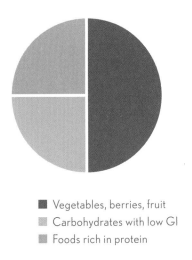

■ Vegetables, berries, fruit
▦ Carbohydrates with low GI
▨ Foods rich in protein

1. Vegetables, fruits, and berries are essential for your health and should be regarded as the main constituent of the meal—so they get half your plate!

3. Eat protein at every meal—depending on your body size, about 25 to 30 grams per meal. All protein sources are good, but plant protein is in many ways the best due to the accompanying fiber.

2. Starchy accompaniments such as rice, pasta, and potatoes are allowed when eating the Nordic Way, but the total quantity should be only about two-thirds of the volume of the protein. Be sure to choose whole-grain products with a low GI. Consult the chart on page 49.

Of course, you don't need to slavishly follow the plate model every time you eat, but it is an easy guiding principle, especially when you are eating out. Below, we have put together a range of examples of different meals for a day's diet with a high protein content and fewer carbohydrates (and with a lower GI) than normal—that is, a day's diet that meets the ratio 1:2. There are many more examples and inspiration in the recipes, which start on page 69.

Breakfast

- Skyr or plain Greek yogurt with berries and sugar-free muesli, served with a little whole-grain crispbread with low-fat cheese and an orange
- Steel-cut oatmeal with apple and cinnamon, served with a smoothie made with reduced fat or fat-free plain Greek yogurt
- Slice of low-GI bread with ham and a fried egg, served with a latte made with low-fat milk

Morning Snack

- Vegetable sticks dipped in a little hummus
- A small handful of nuts
- Protein bar

Lunch

- Sandwich made with low-GI bread with lean meat or chicken, salad greens, and pickles
- Coleslaw with lemon, honey, feta, and chicken
- Low-GI bread with a serving of hummus, smoked salmon, and fresh spinach

Afternoon Snack

- Cottage cheese with bell peppers and celery
- Smoothie of berries and reduced-fat or fat-free Greek yogurt
- Latte made with low-fat milk

Dinner

- Turkey stir-fry with vegetables and whole-grain pasta, served with avocado salad with feta cheese and snap peas
- Omelet with chicken, asparagus, and tomatoes, served with a green salad
- Fillet of fish with beet salad

Note: We recommend drinking water rather than other beverages (wine, beer, soft drinks, etc.) with meals. Most of us become thirsty during a meal because during the process of digestion, a large volume of enzymes and other fluids leaves the blood and tissues and enters the lumen of the intestine. Eventually, you'll reabsorb most of this solution back into the body, but in the meantime, it's okay to drink water if you're thirsty. In fact, you can always count on your normal thirst mechanisms to tell you when you need to drink and how much.

YOUR NEW BEST FRIENDS: SKYR AND RYE

Throughout the recipe section you will see several items that recur frequently, either as a primary ingredient or as an essential accompaniment meant to be served alongside the recipe and is reflected in the nutritional breakdown. These include skyr (the Scandinavian equivalent of Greek yogurt) and dense, whole-kernel rye bread. Because these ingredients will become key building blocks in your new eating plan, we advise stocking up as you begin to transition to the Nordic Way of eating. You will find skyr, (along with hummus and hard-boiled eggs) an easy, efficient, low-fat way to add protein to a meal when the carbs-to-protein ratio is too carb-heavy. Conversely, a slice of hearty whole rye bread is a simple, low-GI way to introduce healthy carbs into a meal of protein and vegetables that also increases satiety.

Skyr is a breakfast staple throughout Scandinavia that is becoming more widely available in the US; 150 grams (about 5.5 ounces) has just 100 calories and typically 17 grams of protein, equivalent to Greek yogurt. It is also a handy, protein-rich way to add a creamy quality to sauces, dressings, salads, and desserts. Some brands you may find in your grocery store include Siggis, Norr Skyr, and Icelandic Provisions. Always choose plain, unflavored skyr, as fruit and other flavorings invariably add both carbs and calories to this otherwise virtuous product. If you want to sweeten your skyr if you are eating it on its own, better to stir in a teaspoon of honey.

Low-GI whole-kernel (or whole-grain) rye and pumpernickel breads are another traditional Scandinavian favorite, and they are the breads we endorse for our eating plans, too. We are not talking about the soft, fluffy rye bread you might get at a diner or deli; those are made primarily with refined wheat flour and just a little rye flour (as well as coloring). Instead, these European-style breads are close-textured and dense, thinly sliced, and visibly full of cracked or "kibbled" grains. The color ranges from dark golden brown to nearly black. These breads are toothsome and filling, not just "filler." You may need to seek these out online or from a specialty or health-food store, and always check the ingredient list to be sure the first and primary ingredient is whole rye grains and/ or flour. Some brands that offer whole-grain rye breads include Mestemacher, Feldkamp, and Genuine Bavarian. Another alternative that is low-GI although not rye-based is Ezekial 4:9 bread, which is found in the freezer section of many natural-food stores and some supermarkets.

Other items in the Nordic pantry worth seeking out include omega-rich canned fish such as sardines and mackerel, canned chickpeas, nuts like almonds and hazelnuts, rye berries and flakes, low-GI tortillas, and low-GI basmati rice.

WHY DO WE RECOMMEND
LOW-FAT DAIRY PRODUCTS?

Many observational studies are suggesting that there's not much difference in cardiovascular or diabetes risk in people consuming full-fat dairy products versus those eating reduced-fat versions. However, no study is suggesting that butter, cream, and cheese can be eaten with complete abandon. We are guided by the evidence-based science of the DiOGenes study. The food plan that was associated with best outcomes in terms of weight control and cardiovascular risk had 30 percent of its calories from fat, less than 10 percent of that in the form of saturated fat. By reducing carbohydrate intake slightly, we have generally increased intake of protein. Some of those carbs could certainly be replaced by healthy fat like that from nuts, almonds, avocado, canola and olive oil, as well as cheese and full-fat fermented dairy products. However, we recommend that you follow the principles from DiOGenes, which puts a priority on foods like fish, chicken, pork, and eggs because they are such excellent sources of protein. To juggle the ratio of protein to carbohydrate and still stay within your budget of fat, we recommend you choose lower-fat dairy and meat products.

MORE ON WHOLE GRAINS

"Choose whole grains first." This slogan is well known everywhere, but the problem is it doesn't distinguish between finely ground whole grains and actual intact whole grains, even though they have vastly different effects in your body. Let us be clear right away: Although all whole grains are better than refined ones, *intact* whole-grain products are by far the best choice. They are more likely to be lower GI and therefore good for your satiety and weight, and they can also help prevent cardiovascular diseases and certain forms of cancer.

The differences—and health issues—between finely ground whole grains and visible-to-the-naked-eye whole or cracked grains are due to the different ways they affect blood glucose. Breads made from very finely ground whole-grain flour increase blood glucose as fast and strongly as white bread—in other words, they are high GI even though they are whole grain. And that is neither desirable for your energy level nor your desire for sweets. Low-GI whole grains, on the other hand, are in a league of their own.

New research from the University of Lund in Sweden has compared the satiety from whole and ground barley grains, respectively. After a serving of whole, boiled barley grains for dinner, the satiety lasted up to sixteen hours. This means a lower calorie intake during breakfast and lunch the next day. If the barley grains, on the other hand, were ground to flour, the feeling of satiety decreased. It was a very clear, strong effect and doesn't only apply to barley, but to other types of grains such as wheat and oats.

The reason for such a big difference between real intact whole grains and flour made from them is that the body's digestive processes really have to work (hard) when intact whole grains are to be broken down. The shell around the grains is full of tough dietary fiber that protects the rest of the grain and takes extra long to digest. When the grains are ground the nutrients are absorbed far faster, which results in a poorer long-term satiety. And the blood glucose increases more rapidly and subsequently drops. These roller coaster rides drain you of energy, make you hungry, and can increase the risk of lifestyle diseases.

Therefore, our recommendation is clear: as often as possible, you should choose cereal products in which the percentage of whole grains is the biggest and on top of that aim for grains that have the grain itself intact.

FOODS HIGH IN PROTEIN

ANIMAL SOURCES	GRAMS PER 100G
Lean beef	21.6
Lean lamb	20.4
Lean chicken	20.4
Lean turkey	21.9
Lean pork	21.6
White fish (average)	21.1
Salmon (fresh)	20.2
Salmon (canned)	21.9
Salmon (smoked)	25.4
Sardines (canned in oil)	23.7
Tuna (canned)	22.8
Prawns	22.6
Oysters	10.8
Scallops	23.2
Cheese (parmesan)	35.1
Cheese (cheddar)	25.4
Cottage cheese	13.6
Yogurt	Range 5 to 8
Milk, low-fat	3.7
Egg	13.2 (about 6g per egg)
PLANT SOURCES	
Almonds, raw	16.9
Almond butter	8.8
Brazil nuts	12.0
Peanuts	24.3
Peanut butter	22.6
Cashews	15.3
Walnuts	15.4
Lentils	7.6
Chickpeas	8.0
Hummus	7.7
Baked beans in tomato sauce	5.1
Tofu	7.9

GLYCEMIC INDEX (GI) VALUES OF COMMON CARBOHYDRATE FOODS

Foods with a GI of 55 or less are classed as low-GI foods. Foods with a GI of 70 or more are considered high-GI. Foods with a moderate GI (56–69) are intermediate but they can still contribute to lowering the average GI of your diet, particularly if used in place of a high-GI counterpart with a GI above 80.

HIGH CARBOHYDRATE FOODS			
White bread	70–75	White rice	73
Whole wheat bread (fine*)	74	Brown rice	68
Unleavened wheat bread	68	Barley	28
Black rye bread (fine*)	76	Sweet corn	52
Light rye bread	68	Spaghetti, white	49
Whole-grain rye bread (coarse*)	46–62	Spaghetti, whole wheat	48
Pumpernickel	50	Rice noodles	53
Corn tortilla	46	Couscous	65
DAIRY PRODUCTS AND ALTERNATIVES			
Milk, full-fat	27–31	Yogurt, low-fat plain	20–35
Milk, non-fat	30–34	Soy milk	34
Ice cream, low fat vanilla	36	Rice milk	92
BREAKFAST CEREALS			
Cornflakes	81	All-Bran	50
Shredded wheat	75	Bran flakes	74
Steel-cut oats	52	Muesli	40
Instant oatmeal	79		
VEGETABLES**			
Green peas	51	Potato, french-fried	63
Sweet corn	46	Carrots, steamed	39
Potato, russet	85	Sweet potato, baked	46–65
Potato, Carisma™	53	Butternut squash	51
Potato, instant	97		
LEGUMES (CANNED)			
Chickpeas	28	Soybeans	16
Kidney beans	24	Baked beans	49
Lentils	32		

FRUIT AND FRUIT PRODUCTS			
Apple	36	Peaches, canned	43
Orange	43	Strawberry jam/jelly	49
Banana	51	Apple juice	41
Pineapple	59	Orange juice	50
Watermelon#	76	Golden raisins	56
Dates	39–45	Raisins	56
Prunes	40		
SUGARS			
Agave syrup	19	Maple-flavored syrup	68
Table sugar	65	Corn syrup	90
Maple syrup, pure	49	Honey	61
SNACK PRODUCTS			
Chocolate, plain	45	Corn chips	74
Chocolate, dark	23	Soft drink/soda	59
Potato chips	56	Rice crackers	87

GI values can be searched online at www.glycemicindex.com.

The Shoppers Guide to GI Values by Jennie Brand-Miller and Kaye Foster-Powell (Da Capo, 2015) is a handy pocket book.

Breads marked with an asterisk (*) are made from finely milled 100% flours in which the fiber is retained but finely ground. They include the micronutrients of the original grain but are digested rapidly because the starch is fully gelatinized. When you can see densely packed whole kernels in the bread, chances are its low GI.

Watermelon and other melons have a high GI but they are also very low in carbohydrates. This means they have a low glycemic load and you can still include them in your healthy low-GI diet. Strawberries and other berries also have a very low carbohydrate content. You should eat as much as you wish.

** The majority of green, red, yellow and orange vegetables have a low carbohydrate content too (and very few calories). This means they have a low glycemic load and they pack a punch when it comes to micronutrients. You SHOULD include them in a healthy low-GI diet. In contrast, the starchy vegetables such as potatoes and sweet potatoes contain a lot of carbohydrates. Most varieties of potato have a very high GI, but in Australia we are beginning to see low-GI varieties such as Carisma™ on the market.

By this point we hope you have been convinced that eating according to the precepts of the Nordic Way and its golden 2:1 ratio will help you curb the desire to overeat, and maintain a healthy weight. But the benefits don't stop there.

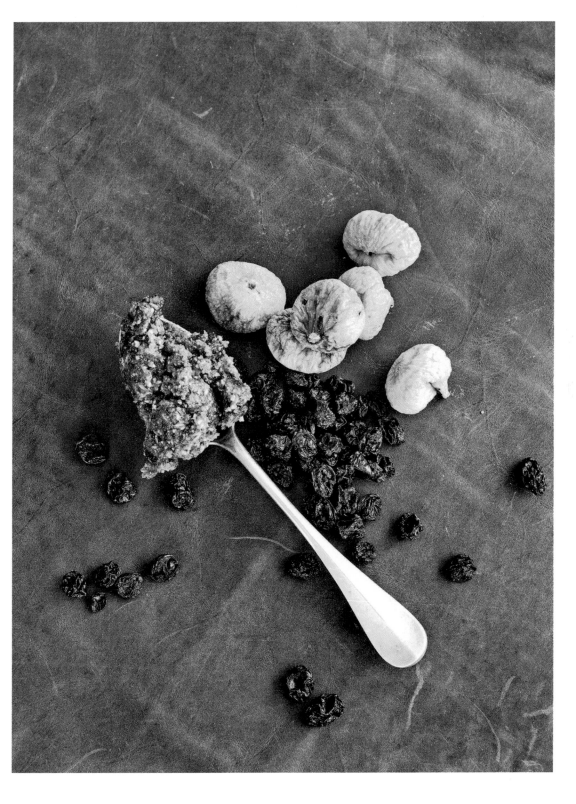

A FLATTER STOMACH

Many people struggle to lose weight around their stomach, and this has led to the rise of many questionable "flat stomach" diets, along with liposuction and plastic surgery. Fortunately, all you have to do to make your stomach shrink is combine the right foods with exercise. A large stomach is often caused by a combination of excess fat under the skin, a lax abdominal wall, and too much fat around the organs in the abdomen.

A lax abdominal wall is especially seen in women who have given birth, but it is actually applicable to most people over thirty who do not regularly exercise their abdominal muscles. So the easiest gain is obtained by doing core abdominal exercises for just a few minutes every day. Doing 1-minute planks regularly can work wonders!

The next step is regular physical activity, because this will also quite effectively reduce the amount of fat in the abdominal wall. Do this two or three times a week, pushing the heart rate up, so that half the time the heart rate should get up so high that you cannot talk at the same time. It can be anything from Zumba to jogging to Peak 8s to any other activities that make you sweat. Several studies suggest that it is easier to keep going if you train with others, but of course it has to fit into your everyday life.

Moreover, we recommend that you drink water with your meals rather than alcohol. Having water before and during meals increases satiety and makes it easier to consume less calories without conscious effort. So save the alcoholic beverages for cocktail hour and not the dinner table.

THE NORDIC WAY WILL HELP YOU GET A FLAT STOMACH!

Besides exercise, *The Nordic Way* has an entirely independent stomach-slimming effect due to the protein content of the diet. And if you want to turbo-charge it, you should make sure that every meal of the day has the right protein ratio. You will speed it up further by eating more dairy protein especially. If you include foods such as Greek yogurt (with higher protein content) or, even better, skyr, lower-fat cheese (e.g., cottage cheese), and low-fat milk, you will boost your weight loss around the stomach. We do not really know why dairy products seem to be better for abdominal fat loss than other protein-rich foods, such as fish, meat, and beans, but several studies point in that direction. If you do not tolerate or wish to eat dairy products, don't worry. You'll still see a great effect on your abdominal fat if you just eat according to the diet's principles.

Part of the fat inside the abdominal wall will be burned and disappear when you exchange carbohydrates with protein, which is precisely what you do when you eat *The Nordic Way*. But you can speed up the process further by avoiding fruit juice and soft drinks and drinking milk instead. In the experiments we have carried out in collaboration with Professor Bjørn Richelsen from Aarhus University, Denmark, we found that overweight individuals who drank low-fat milk instead of cola (for the same number of calories) lost a lot of fat inside the abdomen. You could achieve the same outcome by substituting a protein drink made from whey, pea, or rice protein if drinking milk doesn't appeal. The sugary drink increased the abdominal fat of the overweight individuals, while the milk made the abdominal fat shrink. The results are published in the *American Journal of Clinical Nutrition* and have attracted great attention around the world.

FOUR WAYS TO A FLATTER STOMACH

1. Abdominal exercises for strengthening the abdominal muscles
2. Fitness training for reducing abdominal fat
3. *The Nordic Way* with an optimal protein content in all the meals of the day
4. Exchanging drinks rich in sugar for drinks with protein (eg skim milk)

HOW MUCH FAT
DO YOU HAVE
ON YOUR BODY?

In a hectic and busy everyday life, it can be hard to live healthy and take care of your weight. An important precondition for your success is that you set a realistic goal for the weight at which you stabilize. What is realistically possible? And how slim do you really want to be? Some people have unrealistic ambitions of reaching a weight that will require them to think about every bite they eat, which of course has consequences for quality of life. There is no magic body mass index (BMI) that is right for everyone. A healthy and lean body is about finding the balance that works for you.

BMI is a useful general index for assessing body weight status—under 25 is healthy, 25 to 30 is overweight, and 30+ is obese. However, BMI does not give a truthful picture of how much fat you have on your body, which is what matters. Fitness centers offer fat measurements with various instruments that measure the conductivity of the body by sending a mild current through the feet and hands. The measurements give an approximate estimate of the body fat mass but only because of the equation they contain—which you can use at home for free! If you have a calculator, this is how you do it:

MALE:
Fat mass (lbs) = (0.66 * weight (lbs)) - (0.66 * height (cm)) - (0.044 * age) + 43.6

FEMALE:
Fat mass (lbs) = (0.66 * weight (lbs)) - (0.66 * height (cm)) - (0.044 * age) + 68.6

Example:
A 55-year-old woman weighs 165 lbs and is 165 cm tall.

Fat mass (lbs) = (0.66 × 165)–(0.66 × 165 cm)–(0.044 × 55) + 31.2

Remember to multiply the numbers inside the brackets before they are put together and subtracted. The fat mass is: 108.9–108.9–2.4 + 68.6 = 66 lbs.

This means that 66 lbs out of the 165 lbs is fat.

It can be a good thing to know how much fat you have on your body, but you would probably also like to know what is normal. It is just hard to say, since it is dependent on sex, age, and height. Therefore, it is more suitable to calculate the fat percentage of the body, which is the percentage of fat of your total weight.

Fat mass (lbs) × 100 =

The fat percentage of the body =

Weight (lbs)

In the example above you insert the fat mass and weight:

66 lbs × 100

The fat percentage of the body = 40%

Minor overweight is defined as a body fat percentage between 20 and 25 percent for men and between 30 and 35 percent for women, while actual overweight is when the body fat percentage exceeds 25 percent for men and 35 percent for women.

You should be aware that if the BMI is lower than 25 or 26, the formula will often give a too-high body fat percentage. So if your weight is low, it is better to only use BMI, waist girth, and of course the mirror! When your BMI is between 18.5 and 25, which indicates that you are slim, you should consider whether it is because you have a lot of muscle and maybe strong bones, or if you, despite your normal BMI, perhaps still have too much fat on your body. In this case, the mirror is actually a better measure than expensive machines, scanners, or formulas!

Even if your body fat percentage is high, it is not necessarily very harmful to your health. If the fat is in the "right" places, that is, on the legs, hips, and thighs (pear shape), it is not as harmful as if it is wrapped around the stomach (apple shape), that is, around the vital organs. The health-related benefits of losing weight are definitely highest if you tend to carry weight around your midsection.

IS ALCOHOL HEALTHY?

You can skip this section if you do not drink alcohol, because no one should start drinking beer or wine in order to achieve health gains. But if you enjoy a glass or two now and then, read on.

Perhaps you have heard that wine is healthier than beer because of a range of beneficial antiaging chemicals in wine, and maybe you even use it as an argument for drinking three or four glasses in one night. The only problem is that research has documented that it takes a minimum of fourteen glasses of wine a day in order to get enough of the health-promoting substances! That is simply too much alcohol and will damage your body instead.

WHAT DO WE KNOW?

Several population studies, including a large Danish study, have shown that individuals who prefer wine have a lower risk of cardiovascular diseases than individuals who prefer beer. That makes it sound like wine is healthier, but when researchers examined all the population studies from around the world, moderate amounts of beer and wine were equally healthy. In some countries, wine drinkers generally live more healthfully than beer drinkers —it's *not* the alcohol or wine but other things in their lives, such as a healthier diet and more physical activity, that drives the benefit. In other words, wine is not healthier than beer, but moderate consumption of beer and wine is related to the same reduction of the risk of diabetes, cardiovascular diseases, and dementia. This is because alcohol increases the HDL cholesterol of the blood, decreases blood clotting, and increases insulin sensitivity. Does that mean you can have a drink? Absolutely. Just stick to moderate amounts and you will come out on the right side of health.

HOW MUCH IS TOO MUCH?

A simple rule of thumb, if you drink, is up to one drink a day for women and up to two for men. Larger amounts increase the risk of a range of lifestyles diseases, such as overweight and cancer, so a moderate consumption is prudent. It is also worth knowing that the health benefits of moderate alcohol are increased if you spread your consumption out evenly over the week rather than having many drinks on, say, the weekend!

BEER OR WINE?

Even though wine has had so much good press, several factors actually point toward beer being a little healthier: A regular beer has 45 percent fewer calories per 100 mL than wine, and about 60 percent lower alcohol density. In addition, beer contains a range of B vitamins that are beneficial to health. And if you choose a light beer or an alcohol-free beer, you will get even fewer calories, with almost the same good taste.

HERBS AND SPICES

Herbs and spices are routinely praised as miracle remedies that can cure everything from cancer and nausea to a broken heart. These sensational stories originate in everything from test tube studies to ancient alternative medical principles.

The bottom line is that herbs and spices contain a range of phytochemicals that might have an impact on our health. In the plants, their biological functions are meant to protect against the sun's ultraviolet radiation and attacks from rodents, fungus, and bacteria. The harsher the conditions in which the herbs are grown, the more phytochemicals they will contain. Some may be nutritious but some may not be—naturally occurring toxicants consumed in large amounts have been known to have adverse effects in humans and animals (e.g., goitrogens).

Yet most of us consume herbs and spices in such small amounts that it will hardly have any great health-related significance. They taste wonderful, of course, because they add lots of aroma and complexity to many dishes. We use the fresh ones in abundance in our recipes, but you should find your own balance and not feel compelled to eat them for health reasons.

Our planet has limited resources and humans are currently taxing those to the limit. Paleo diets and other programs that are based on a *very large* intake of protein and very little carbohydrate are pushing the envelope.

But new research shows that greenhouse gas emissions generated by raising some forms of meat, such as pork and poultry, are substantially lower than they are for beef. In fact, per calorie, pork, chicken, and eggs have a similar environmental impact to fruit and vegetables. Moreover, many of the fish that we recommend in our recipes—those most commonly used in the Scandinavian countries—are plentiful and sustainable. Sardines, mackerel, and organically farmed salmon are all good options that do not endanger the health of our oceans.

In short, because our food plan is based on *modestly* higher protein intake and a moderate carbohydrate intake from plant foods, by helping you to maintain a lower and healthy weight for life, you are reducing your carbon footprint and doing your best for both yourself and for future generations.

PROTEIN MAKES YOU BRIGHTER

It's true—high-protein diets are good for mental function! A three-week experiment in Arne's lab involving young males on a protein-rich diet showed a dramatic improvement in their mental performance. Twenty-three men between nineteen and thirty-one years were divided into two groups. The first group continued with their usual protein intake, while the second group consumed twice as much protein, mostly from milk and meat, for three weeks. A computer-based test showed that the number of mistakes decreased and the speed of submitting the correct answers improved among the second group. Moreover, the test subjects did better on a test of orientation that involved simple questions on time and place. The improvement in brain function could be explained by an increased content of certain protein building blocks in the blood, so-called amino acids, which increased concurrently with the raised protein consumption. These amino acids are believed to be able to increase the content of neurotransmitters in the brain, which lead to faster reactions in the brain. Earlier studies were only one day long, so this study was the first to prove the important impact of a long-term increase in protein consumption. Most public dietary recommendations on calories, fat, carbohydrates, and protein focus on preventing obesity, diabetes, and cardiovascular diseases. Hopefully, this study can help set the record straight and put preserving mental function on the map as an important benefit of higher-protein diets.

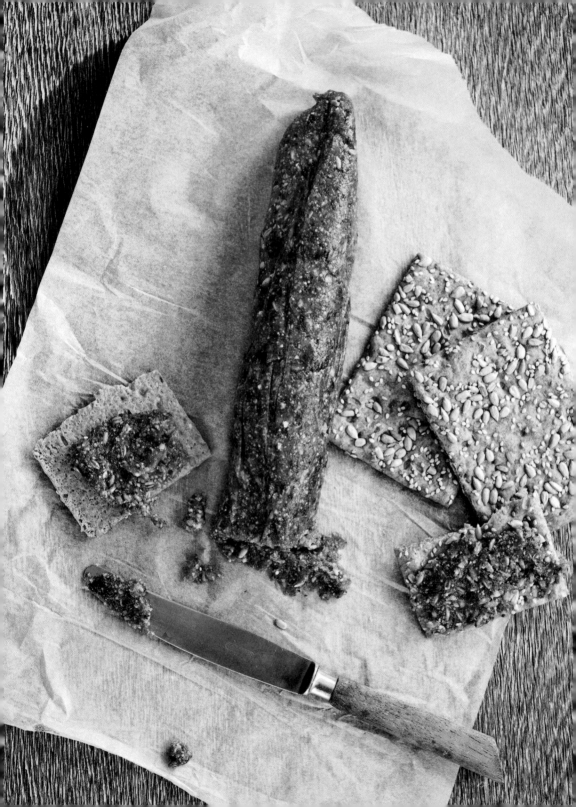

PART 3

EATING THE NORDIC WAY: MEAL PLANS AND RECIPES

NOW IT IS TIME TO MOVE PAST THE THEORECTICAL STAGE AND TO START ASSEMbling meals that hit that sweet spot of 2:1 carbs to protein. If you are not quite that comfortable applying the principles of the Nordic Way on your own, no worries; we have put together a four-week plan that can serve as a blueprint for your new eating style.

Although *The Nordic Way* is constructed to minimize hunger and deprivation, you may find that your body "reacts" to the new diet. You might experience hunger, fatigue, uneasiness in the body, and perhaps worse sleep quality for a few days. These are entirely normal reactions when you eat differently from how you usually do. Think of it as your body doing spring cleaning. It is usually not much fun while you are in it, but the joy and the feeling of a clean house (in this case, your body) is amazing. So hang in there. It is *not* easy changing the way you eat, because unhealthy temptations, dinner parties with friends, and the old habits are waiting in the wings to undermine your good intentions.

Let the first four weeks of weight control be devoted to your *well-being*. This is the time for you to show yourself and your body that you are serious about this and that the natural effect of healthy food and exercise on the body will continue. It might as well get used to it! We promise it will not take long before your body will love you for it, and you will love the feeling of energy and well-being that will course through your body—not to mention the nice numbers on your bathroom scale that prove you are keeping unwanted pounds at bay!

Prioritize preparing the healthy, simple food from the meal plans and try to keep these first weeks as simple as possible. Don't schedule twenty dinner dates with guests or activities away from home. You need to be persistent in putting yourself and your body's needs first while you get used to your new life. These healthy changes will slowly turn into habits if you give them time to do so. And your investment in your health will be repaid many times over.

Think about other things you have accomplished in your life—many of which were more challenging than simply making some alterations in the way you combine foods!—and believe that you can do this as well! After the first couple of weeks you will see big results and it will get easier.

Follow the plans on pages 64–67 as closely as possible, although you should feel free to interchange days and meals, even from earlier weeks.

All the recipes from the plan can be found in the book, but our appetites are different. It is important that you spend the next four weeks becoming acquainted with your hunger and satiety! The portions for all of our recipes are generous, but they are simply guidelines. Our recommendation is that you "eat to appetite," which means you should eat *just* until you are no longer hungry, not until you are stuffed.

If you are still very hungry after eating a full portion, wait a little bit before augmenting your meal. Your hunger regulation may just need a little time to work. Remember that your meals should be divided with about half vegetables (preferably the coarse ones, such as cabbage, broccoli, etc.), 120 to 180g lean meat or fish depending on your size, and a similar volume (or less) of a low-GI carb such as pasta, basmati rice, or whole-grain bread. It is also okay to do without the pasta, rice, etc., and eat only the meat or fish and vegetables, if you want to save space for dessert!

For these first days on the eating plan, you may find it easiest to monitor your carb-to-protein intake if you eat most of your meals at home, or prepare meals at home to take along with you for breakfast and/or lunch if you work outside the home. If you do not have the opportunity to pack a homemade lunch during the week, you can certainly put together something from a salad bar, but keep the following four rules in mind:

- Pile up the veggies first and stay away from the prepared white carbs like rice salad.

- Don't skimp on the protein from meat, fish, eggs, and so on.

- Chickpeas and other legumes are a good low-GI carb to enjoy as a side.

- Drink water with every meal.

After enjoying the four weeks of *The Nordic Way* menus, you should have a feeling of what works the best for you and what does not work. You cannot be on a "diet" for the rest of your life, so your new healthy habits should fit you and not the other way around. Do what works best for you, your family, and your everyday life. Remember, nothing is prohibited; it's all about balancing the things you love and don't want to give up (namely carbs and sweets) with things that feed your body what it needs (lean proteins and plant foods). You can always come back to the menus if you feel the need to get back on the straight and narrow, but we're confident that after a few weeks of following our plan, you will get the hang of it and can start to convert your own favorite menus and recipes to *The Nordic Way*.

MENUS

DAY	BREAKFAST	SNACK	LUNCH	SNACK	DINNER
Monday	Crispbread with egg and cottage cheese (page 83)	1 carrot, cut into sticks, with your choice of dip (page 228)	Quinoa with roast beef, tomato, and watercress (page 110)	15 almonds	Omelet with mackerel, tomatoes, and rye bread (page 181)
Tuesday	Hot cereal "to go" (page 69)	100 grams grapes	Meatballs with edamame and cabbage (page 138)	1 slice toasted rye with your choice of dip (page 228)	Salmon with herbs, quick cucumber pickle, and egg (page 182)
Wednesday	Skyr with granola (page 72)	1 apple, sliced, with your choice of dip (page 228)	Two-bread sandwich (page 129)	100 grams grapes	Edamame with cabbage and dill (page 165)
Thursday	Fried egg with almond butter sandwich (page 79)	1 pear, sliced, with your choice of dip (page 228)	Rye salad with lemon and berries (page 121)	Roasted chickpeas and almonds (page 91)	Chicken breast with pears, grapes, and rice (page 137)
Friday	Egg white omelet with peppers and cheese (page 84)	15 almonds	Soba noodles with tofu, ginger, and sugar snaps (page 118)	1 carrot, cut into sticks, with your choice of dip (page 228)	Chicken salad (page 117)
Saturday	Bircher muesli (page 87)	1 carrot with your choice of dip (page 228)	Rye berries with cucumber and hazelnuts (page 114)	1 slice low-GI bread with avocado-chocolate spread (page 202)	Chicken with carrots and potatoes (page 189)
Sunday	Pita with ham, carrot, and cottage cheese (page 76)	Crispy kiwifruit (page 108)	Beggar's purses with hummus and cottage cheese (page 130)	1 rye roll with chocolate (page 92)	Pizza with chicken and greens (page 157) or leftovers from the week

DAY	BREAKFAST	SNACK	LUNCH	SNACK	DINNER
Monday	Fried egg with almond butter sandwich (page 79)	1 pear, sliced, with your choice of dip (page 228)	Rice paper rolls with shrimp (page 183)	Low-GI whole-grain bread with avocado-chocolate spread (page 202)	Cod and tomato salad (page 186)
Tuesday	Ham and cheese omelet (page 75)	1 carrot with your choice of dip (page 228)	Tuna, potatoes, and eggs (page 122)	1 rye roll with chocolate (page 92)	Open-faced sandwich with salmon, ginger, and lime (page 145)
Wednesday	Hot cereal "to go" (page 69)	Pita with cottage cheese and apple (page 100)	Chicken, corn, and cornichons (page 126)	15 almonds	Chicken, cabbage, and curry wrap (page 178)
Thursday	Skyr with granola (page 72)	Crispy kiwifruit (page 108)	Egg and vegetables salad on toasted rye (page 133)	1 low-GI whole-grain crispbread bread with your choice of dip (page 228)	Tuna with wasabi, cabbage, almonds, and cucumber (page 158)
Friday	Warm rye cereal with apple and hazelnuts (page 80)	1 pear, sliced, with your choice of dip (page 228)	Chilled tomato soup (page 109)	1 slice low-GI bread with nut butter	Chicken with eggplant, tomato, and cinnamon (page 169)
Saturday	Hot cereal with blueberries (page 71)	Apple with lemon and cocoa nibs (page 103)	Quinoa with roast beef, tomato, and watercress (page 110)	Crunchy egg (page 95)	Salmon meatballs with chickpeas and cabbage (page 162)
Sunday	Sunday morning breakfast (page 88)	1 apple, sliced, with your choice of dip (page 228)	Fennel, prosciutto, and almonds (page 113)	1 slice low-GI bread with almond butter	Chia-crusted tofu with tomato, spinach, and green bean rice (page 170)

WEEK THREE

DAY	BREAKFAST	SNACK	LUNCH	SNACK	DINNER
Monday	Warm rye cereal with apple and hazelnuts (page 80)	1 carrot with your choice of dip (page 228)	Soba noodles with tofu, ginger, and sugar snaps (page 118)	Egg with cottage cheese and almonds (page 99)	Shrimp with chile, grapefruit, and cabbage (page 174)
Tuesday	Bircher muesli (page 87)	Crunchy egg (page 95)	Rye salad with lemon and berries (page 121)	Pear with pepper and mozzarella (page 104)	Salmon with avocado, peas, and fennel (page 142)
Wednesday	Crispbread with egg and cottage cheese (page 83)	1 apple, sliced, with your choice of dip (page 228)	Mackerel, cabbage, and rye bread (page 125)	Carrots with green pea dip (page 96)	Citrus chicken with roasted sweet potato and arugula (page 150)
Thursday	Skyr with granola (page 72)	1 slice toasted low-GI bread with your choice of dip (page 228)	Fennel, prosciutto, and almonds (page 113)	1 grapefruit	Stuffed peppers with lamb, quinoa, and lemon (page 134)
Friday	Hot cereal with blueberries (page 71)	Roasted chickpeas and almonds (page 91)	Chilled tomato soup (page 109)	2 carrot sticks with your choice of dip (page 228)	Fish wontons with cabbage and carrot salad (page 197)
Saturday	Egg white omelet with peppers and cheese (page 84)	1 apple, sliced, with your choice of dip (page 228)	Two-bread sandwich (page 129)	Egg with cottage cheese and almonds (page 99)	Fish fillet with radicchio salad (page 198)
Sunday	Sunday morning breakfast (page 88)	15 almonds	Beggar's purses with hummus and cottage cheese (page 130)	1 grapefruit	Sauté of root vegetables with chorizo (page 173) or leftovers from the week

WEEK FOUR					
DAY	BREAKFAST	SNACK	LUNCH	SNACK	DINNER
Monday	Skyr with granola (page 72)	Apple with lemon and cocoa nibs (page 103)	Rye berries with cucumber and hazelnuts (page 114)	Crispy kiwifruit (page 108)	Chicken drumsticks with fennel and lentils (page 161)
Tuesday	Egg white omelet with peppers and cheese (page 84)	1 carrot with your choice of dip (page 228)	Two-bread sandwich (page 129)	15 almonds	Beef with salt and vinegar potatoes (page 141)
Wednesday	Pita with ham, carrot, and cottage cheese (page 76)	Pear with pepper and mozzarella (page 104)	Quinoa with roast beef, tomato, and watercress (page 110)	Mango, almonds, and mint (page 107)	Pork with sage and halloumi filling (page 146)
Thursday	Warm rye cereal with apple and hazelnuts (page 80)	¼ green cabbage with your choice of dip (page 228)	Rye salad with lemon and berries (page 121)	1 apple with your choice of dip (page 228)	Salmon with crunchy vegetables and celery root cream (page 194)
Friday	Hot cereal "to go" (page 69)	1 slice low-GI bread with avocado-chocolate spread (page 202)	Chicken, corn, and cornichons (page 126)	15 almonds	Pasta Bolognese (page 166)
Saturday	Bircher muesli (page 87)	Pita with cottage cheese and apple (page 100)	Egg and vegetables salad on toasted rye (page 133)	Mango, almonds, and mint (page 107)	Cod with carrot and hazelnuts (page 149)
Sunday	Ham and cheese omelet (page 75)	Carrots with green pea dip (page 96)	Mackerel, cabbage, and rye bread (page 125)	1 apple with your choice of dip (page 228)	Spicy Beef and Noodle Wraps (page 190)

Enough reading about food—now it's time to take this book into the kitchen! We've created easy-to-prepare recipes based on modern Nordic food culture, and each dish has been designed to deliver maximum satisfaction for a minimal amount of calories. While each dish may not necessarily have the ideal 2:1 carb-to-protein ratio on its own, we've included a full nutritional breakdown and carb-to-protein ratio for each recipe so you can still keep your diet in balance. For many of the dishes, you can simply supplement an egg or a spoonful of skyr for additional protein, but all can be mixed and matched so that your entire meal hits the target ratio. We're confident that you'll be pleased with your new healthy and Nordic lifestyle, so enjoy and *velbekomme* (bon appétit!), as we say in Scandinavia.

Hot Cereal "To Go"

SERVES 1

Combine the ingredients at home and add boiling water when you get to the office for an almost instant breakfast. You can even mix up the dry ingredients in bulk to keep in your desk for days when you don't have time to make breakfast; add the berries along with the boiling water. Don't omit the skyr, which contributes protein.

¾ cup old-fashioned rolled oats

4 teaspoons chopped almonds

4 teaspoons fresh or frozen blueberries

1 teaspoon chia seeds

Pinch of ground cinnamon

1 teaspoon stevia, or 1 tablespoon honey or sugar

1 teaspoon finely grated lemon zest

Low-fat plain skyr or Cheater's Skyr (page 231), for serving (optional)

Combine the oats, almonds, blueberries, chia seeds, cinnamon, stevia, and lemon zest in a heatproof container. When you get to work, boil ½ to 1 cup water. Pour it over the ingredients, seal the container, and shake to combine. Set aside to soften for a few minutes. Serve topped with a little skyr, if desired.

RATIO (Carb:Protein) = 2:1

PER SERVING: Calories 170 · Protein 8 g · Carbohydrate 16 g · Fiber n/a g · Fat 9 g · Saturated Fat 1 g · Sodium 3 mg

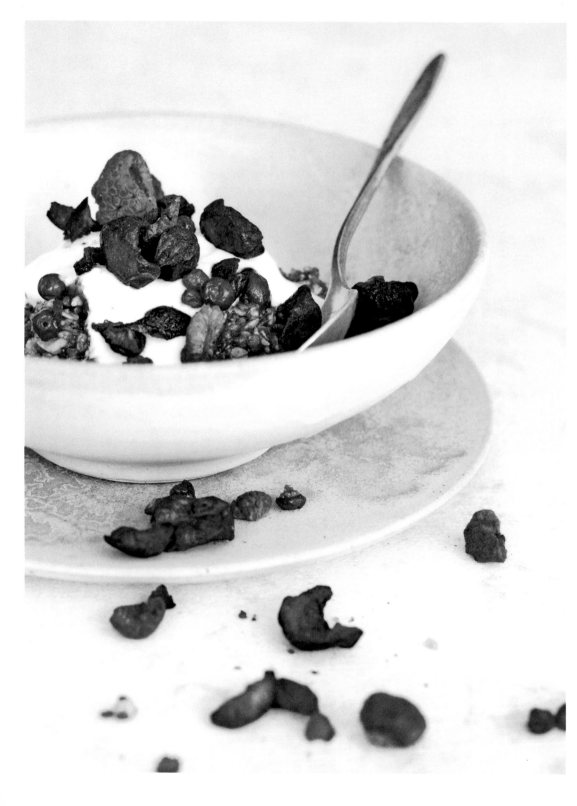

Hot Cereal with Blueberries

SERVES 1

In Denmark, this would be made with just 1 cup water for a toothier texture; try it both ways and see which you like best. Pairing the porridge with an egg gives this breakfast real staying power.

1 cup rolled rye flakes or old-fashioned rolled oats

3 cups cold water

1 egg white

1 apple, cored and grated

½ cup low-fat plain skyr or Cheater's Skyr (page 231)

3 tablespoons fresh or freeze-dried raspberries, blueberries, or raisins

1 large egg, hard-boiled (optional)

Bring the oats, water, and syrup to the boil in a medium saucepan over medium heat. Cook, stirring often, for 5 to 7 minutes, or until the mixture starts to thicken, then reduce the heat to low and cook until creamy, 10 to 15 minutes more. For the last minute add the egg white and stir thoroughly.

Serve the porridge topped with the apple, skyr, and berries, with the hard-boiled egg on the side, if desired.

RATIO (Carb:Protein) = 2:1

PER SERVING: Calories 300 · Protein 23 g · Carbohydrate 36 g · Fiber 5 g · Fat 6 g · Saturated Fat 2 g · Sodium 24

Skyr with Granola

The classic Nordic breakfast, with a bit of an update. Make this your everyday fallback and you'll effortlessly start every morning with the perfect carb-to-protein ratio.

½ cup low-fat plain skyr or
    Cheater's Skyr (page 231)

¼ cup Homemade Granola
    (page 230)

Spoon the skyr into a bowl. Sprinkle the granola on top and serve.

RATIO (Carb:Protein) = 1:3

PER SERVING: Calories 250 · Protein 25 g · Carbohydrate 8 g · Fiber 2 g · Fat 7 g · Saturated Fat 0 g · Sodium 0 mg

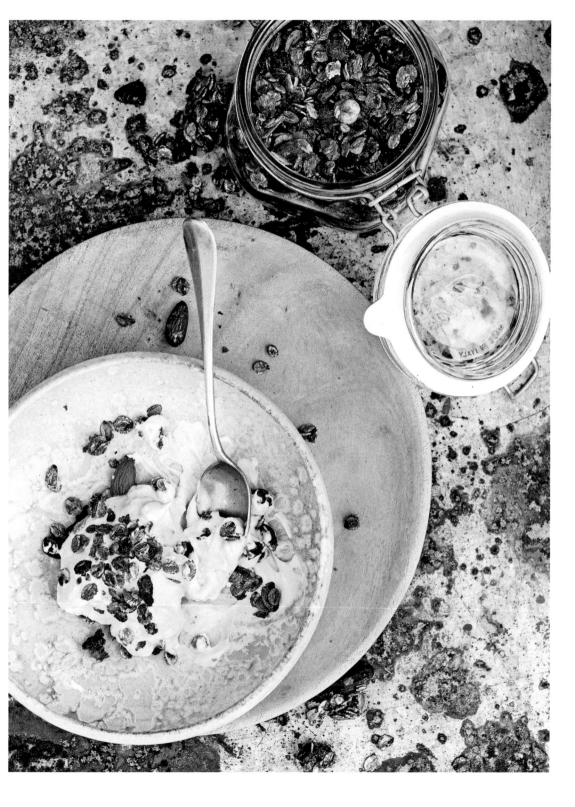

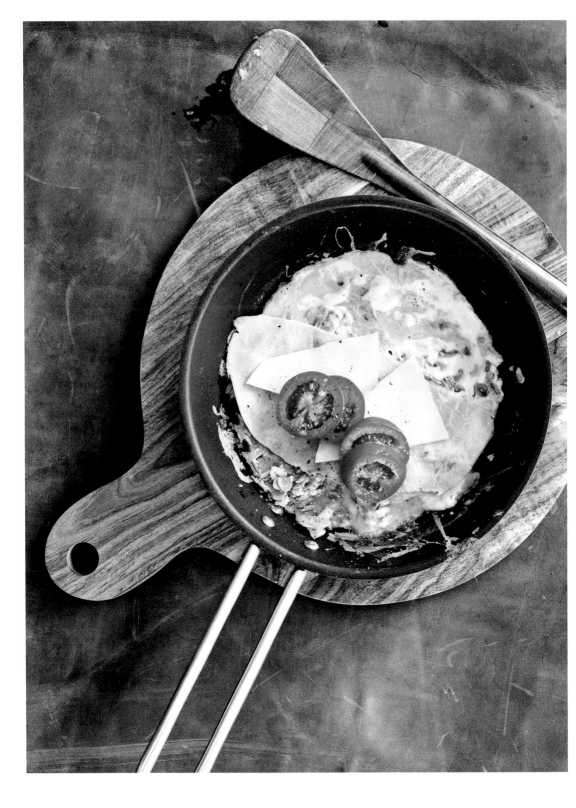

Ham & Cheese Omelet

SERVES 1

With a bit of toasted oats folded into the eggs for body (and carbs), this is a true all-in-one meal. For breakfast on the go, slide the omelet onto parchment paper, add the fillings, and roll it up.

2 large eggs

¼ teaspoon salt

Freshly ground black pepper

1 tablespoon old-fashioned rolled oats

2 teaspoons olive oil

1 slice lean ham

2 slices cheese

1 tomato, sliced

Lightly whisk the eggs with the salt and pepper to taste in a bowl.

Toast the oats in a medium nonstick skillet over medium heat, stirring often, until golden brown, about 3 minutes. Add the oil and then the whisked eggs, tilting the pan so the egg covers the base. Cook for a couple of minutes, or until the egg is just set.

Add the ham, cheese, and tomato. Fold the omelet over the fillings and serve.

RATIO (Carb:Protein) = 2:1

PER SERVING: Calories 440 · Protein 25 g · Carbohydrate 9 g · Fiber 3 g · Fat 34 g · Saturated Fat 15 g · Sodium 689 mg

Pita with Ham, Carrot & Cottage Cheese

SERVES 1

A simple take-along lunch or anytime snack you can make with things you probably have on hand. Carrots add color, crunch, and sweetness.

1 low-GI whole wheat pita bread, lightly toasted

1 teaspoon Dijon mustard

2 slices lean ham

½ carrot, coarsely shredded

¼ cup cottage cheese

Split the pita bread and spread with the mustard. Fill with the ham, carrot, and cottage cheese. Serve.

RATIO (Carb:Protein) = 2:1

PER SERVING: Calories 300 · Protein 22 g · Carbohydrate 36 g · Fiber 6 g · Fat 6 g · Saturated Fat 3 g · Sodium 1,037 mg

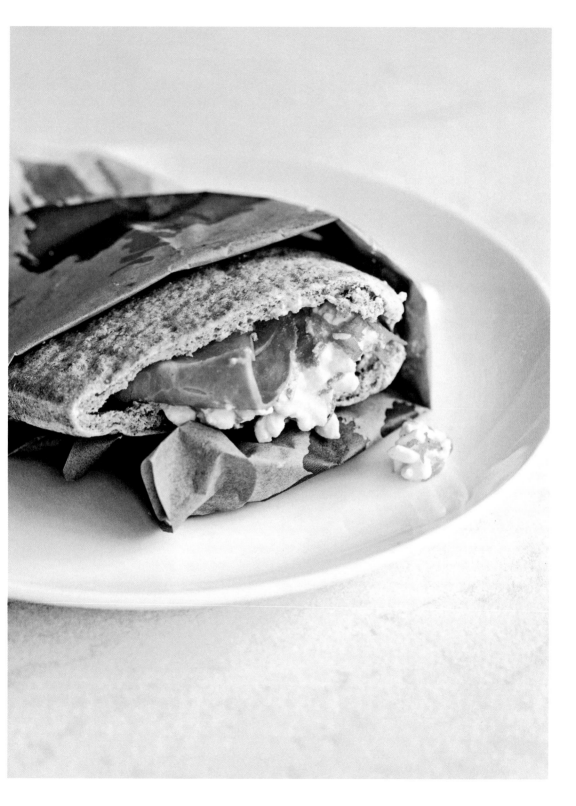

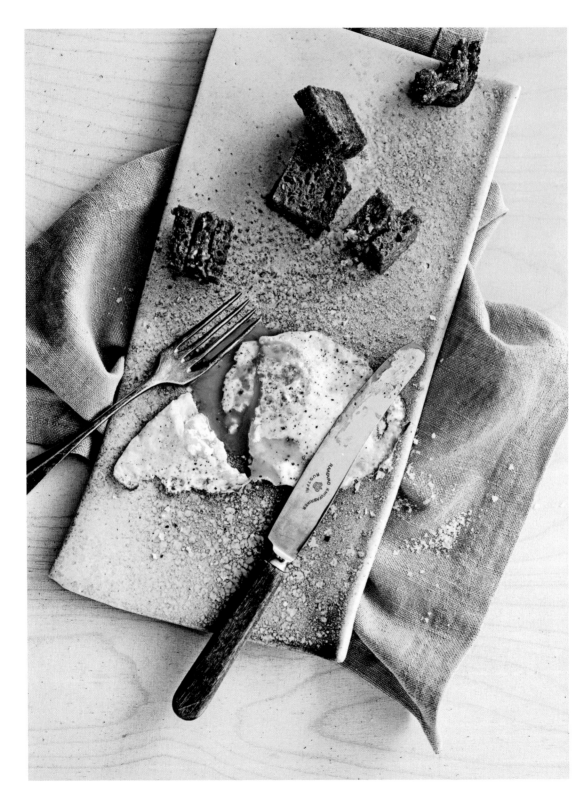

Fried Egg with Almond Butter Sandwich

SERVES 1

This easy breakfast doubles down on protein by pairing a fried egg—an excellent, readily available protein source—with a nut butter sandwich. Choose this for your morning meal when you need something that will keep you going through a demanding day.

4 teaspoons almond butter

1 slice whole-grain rye bread or whole rye pumpernickel bread

Olive oil spray

1 large egg

Spread the nut butter on the bread. Cut the bread in half and sandwich the halves together.

Coat a small nonstick skillet with olive oil spray and heat over medium heat. Add the egg and fry until the white is set, 2 to 3 minutes. Flip the egg, cook for a few more seconds, and transfer to a plate.

Serve the egg with the nut butter sandwich alongside.

RATIO (Carb:Protein) = 3:1

PER SERVING: Calories 290 · Protein 8g · Carbohydrate 27 g · Fiber 4 g · Fat 16 g · Saturated Fat 3 g · Sodium 306 mg

Warm Rye Cereal with Apple & Hazelnuts

SERVES 2

This coarse, rustic style of hot cereal is popular in Denmark. If you prefer a smoother texture, simply triple the liquid quantities and cook until creamy. Thanks to the apple and apple juice, you'll find you won't even be tempted to add sweetener.

1 cup rolled rye flakes or old-fashioned rolled oats

⅔ cup cold water

7 tablespoons apple juice

1 large egg white

½ apple, cored and coarsely shredded (eat the rest of the apple while the cereal is cooking)

2 tablespoons coarsely chopped skinned toasted hazelnuts (see Note)

2 tablespoons low-fat plain skyr or Cheater's Skyr (page 231)

Bring the rye flakes, water, and apple juice to a boil in a medium saucepan over medium heat. Cook over medium-low heat, stirring often, for 5 to 7 minutes, or until the rye flakes are tender. Turn off the heat, stir in the egg white, and set aside for 1 minute. Serve topped with the grated apple, hazelnuts, and skyr.

NOTE: To toast and skin hazelnuts, preheat the oven to 350°F. Spread the nuts on a baking sheet and bake, stirring occasionally, for about 10 minutes, until the skins split. Transfer the nuts to a kitchen towel and let cool for 10 minutes. Use the towel to rub the skins off the nuts. Don't worry if some skin remains. Let cool before chopping.

RATIO (Carb:Protein) = 5:1

PER SERVING: Calories 370 · Protein 11 g · Carbohydrate 52 g · Fiber 7 g · Fat 12 g · Saturated Fat 1 g · Sodium 10 mg

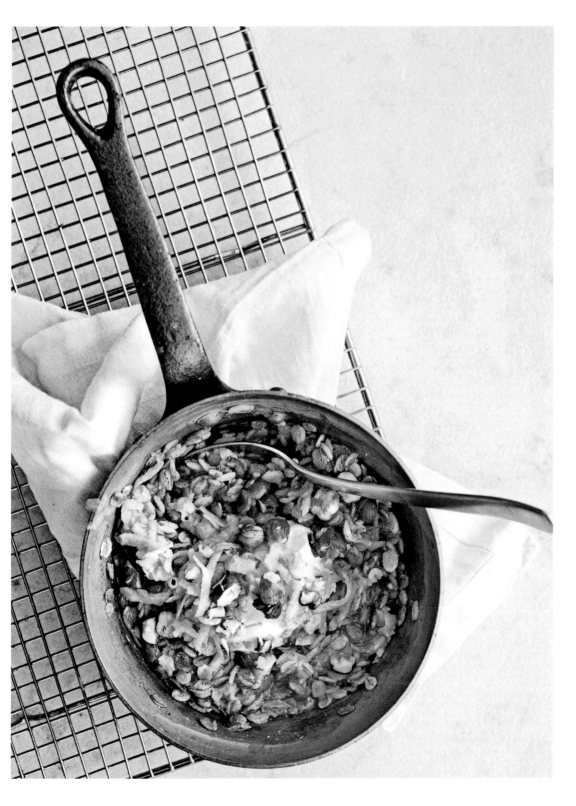

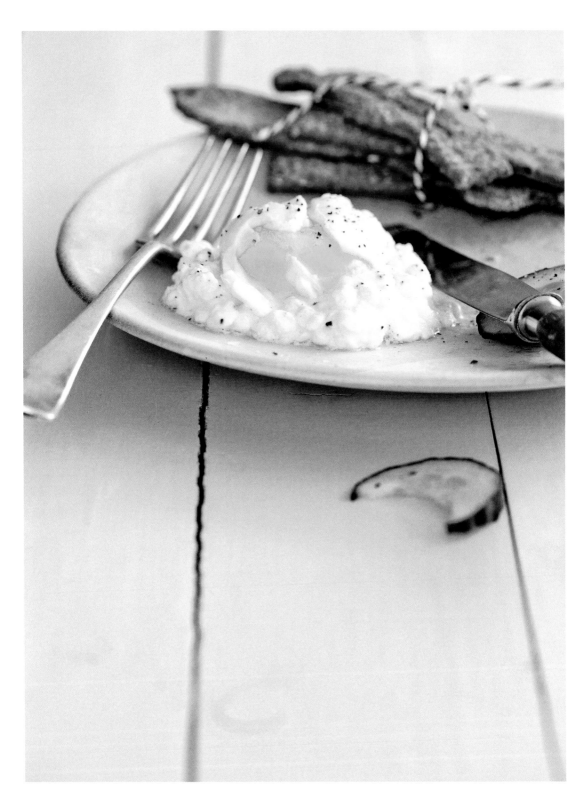

Crispbread with Egg & Cottage Cheese

SERVES 1

2 Crispbread (page 201) or store-bought low-GI whole-grain crispbread

6 slices cucumber

1 large egg, poached or hard-boiled and sliced

2 tablespoons cottage cheese

Freshly ground black pepper

Serve the crispbread topped with the cucumber, egg, and cottage cheese, seasoned with the pepper.

RATIO (Carb:Protein) = 2:1

PER SERVING: Calories 332 · Protein 18 g · Carbohydrate 28 g · Fiber 2 g · Fat 16 g · Saturated Fat 4 g · Sodium 377 mg

Egg White Omelet with Peppers & Cheese

Another great option for breakfast on the go that would also work well for lunch.

2 large egg whites

Salt and freshly ground black pepper

1 tablespoon old-fashioned rolled oats

2 teaspoons olive oil

¼ red bell pepper, seeded and cut into thin strips

¼ yellow bell pepper, seeded and cut into strips

2 tablespoons freshly grated Parmesan cheese

Gently whisk the egg whites with salt and pepper to taste in a bowl. Toast the oats in a medium nonstick skillet over medium heat, stirring often, until golden brown, about 5 minutes. Add the oil and then the whisked egg white, tilting the pan so the egg white covers the bottom. Cook for about 2 minutes. Carefully flip the omelet over and cook for about 2 minutes more, or until the egg white is set. Slide the omelet onto a piece of parchment paper. Add the bell pepper strips and the cheese. Roll up the omelet and cut it in half.

RATIO (Carb:Protein) = 1:2

PER SERVING: Calories 230 · Protein 13 g · Carbohydrate 7 g · Fiber 2 g · Fat 16 g · Saturated Fat 6 g · Sodium 217 mg

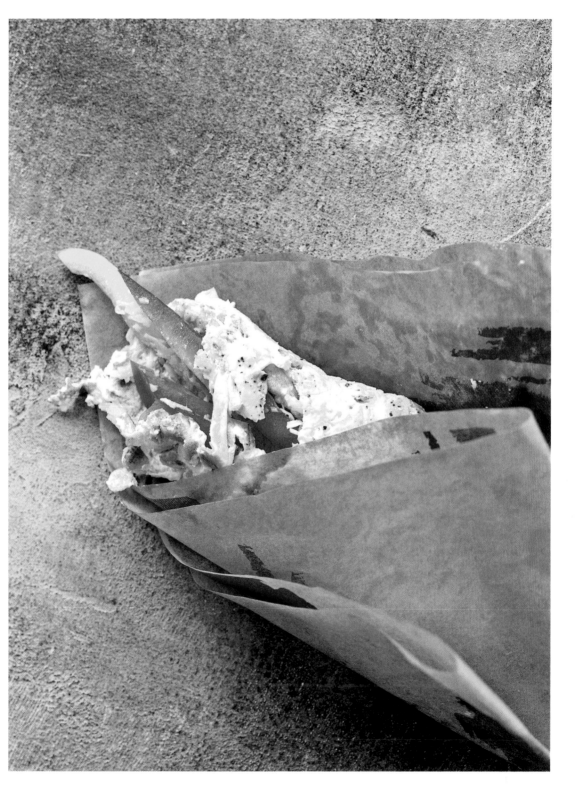

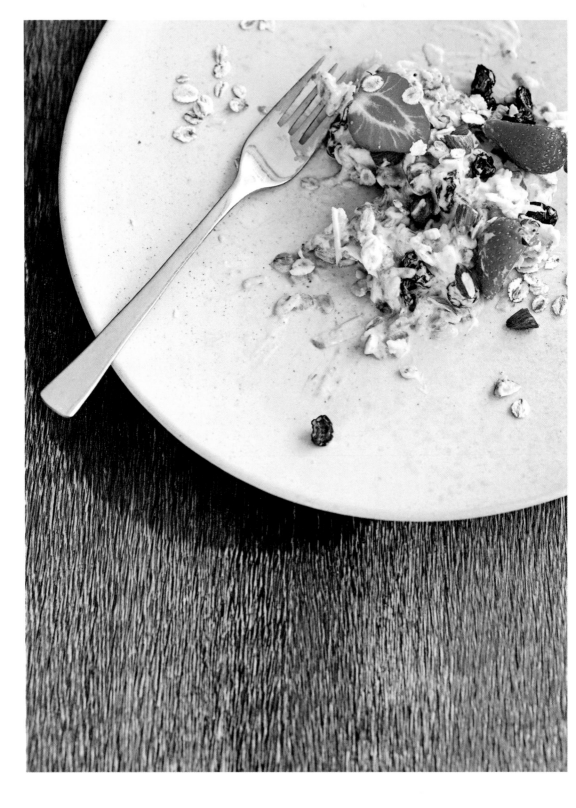

Bircher Muesli

Overnight oats are trendy at the moment, but they have been a staple of the Scandinavian diet for generations. Try our nutty version and see why.

2½ cups old-fashioned rolled oats or rolled rye flakes

Scant 1 cup milk or soy milk, warmed

About ½ cup low-fat plain skyr or Cheater's Skyr (page 231)

2 tablespoons raisins

2 apples, cored and diced, plus ½ apple, cored and shredded

2 handfuls of fresh berries or other seasonal fruit

2 tablespoons chopped almonds

2 tablespoons chopped skinned toasted hazelnuts (see Note, page 80)

2 tablespoons honey

Put the oats in a bowl or jar and pour in the warm milk. Cover and refrigerate overnight. In the morning, add the skyr and mix to combine. If the mixture is too thick, add more skyr. Mix in the raisins, diced apples, and berries, then serve topped with the almonds, hazelnuts, honey, and shredded apple.

RATIO (Carb:Protein) = 5:1

PER SERVING: Calories 480 · Protein 15 g · Carbohydrate 75 g · Fiber 9 g · Fat 12 g · Saturated Fat 2 g · Sodium 34 mg

Sunday Morning Breakfast

SERVES 1

Treat yourself to this smorgasbord of healthy options for a lazy Sunday breakfast in bed.

6 ounces (about 1 cup) chopped or sliced mixed seasonal fruit, as needed

½ cup low-fat plain skyr or Cheater's Skyr (page 231)

1 tablespoon Homemade Granola (page 230) or cocoa nibs

Olive oil spray

1 slice prosciutto or other lean ham

1 large egg

1 slice whole-grain rye bread or whole rye pumpernickel bread

1 tablespoon Hummus (page 206, optional)

Salt and freshly ground black pepper

1 small tomato, sliced

Put the fruit in a glass and top with the skyr and granola.

Spray a medium nonstick skillet with olive oil spray and heat over medium heat. Add the prosciutto and cook until crisp, about 2 minutes. Transfer to a plate. Add the egg to the skillet and cook until the egg is set, about 2 minutes. Flip the egg and cook for a few seconds more. Meanwhile, toast the bread and spread with the hummus (if using). Slide the egg onto the bread and top with the ham. Season with salt and pepper. Serve the open-faced sandwich with the tomato and the fruit salad alongside.

RATIO (Carb:Protein) = 4:3

PER SERVING: Calories 480 · Protein 30 g · Carbohydrate 43 g · Fiber 7 g · Fat 19 g · Saturated Fat 7 g · Sodium 666 mg

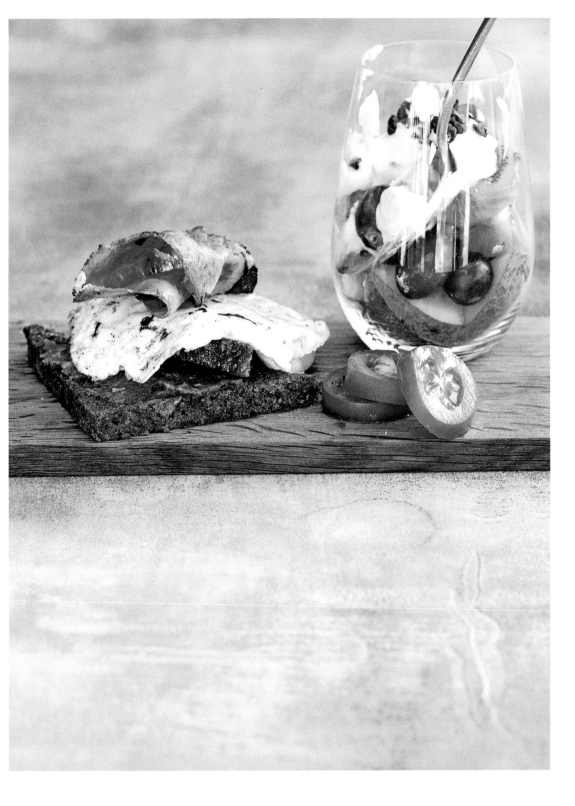

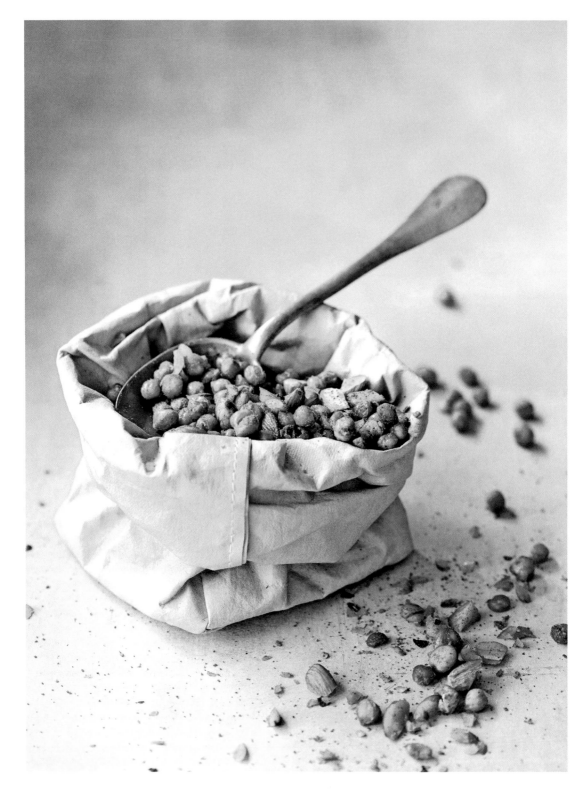

Roasted Chickpeas & Almonds

So much tastier, not to mention healthier, than chips, and just as addictive.

1 cup canned chickpeas, drained
   and rinsed

½ teaspoon paprika

½ teaspoon ground cumin

Pinch of red pepper flakes

Olive oil spray

2 tablespoons coarsely chopped
   raw almonds

Preheat the oven to 325°F. Line a baking sheet with parchment paper.

Spread the chickpeas on paper towels and set aside for 10 minutes to remove any excess moisture. Put the chickpeas in a bowl, add the paprika, cumin, and red pepper flakes, and toss to combine. Spread evenly on the prepared baking sheet and spray lightly with olive oil spray. Roast for 15 minutes, gently shaking the baking sheet after 10 minutes.

Add the almonds, stir to combine, and cook for 10 minutes more, or until the almonds are golden and the chickpeas are slightly crisp. Remove from the oven and cool completely.

Store in an airtight container for up to 1 week.

RATIO (Carb:Protein) = 3:2

PER SERVING: Calories 180 · Protein 8 g · Carbohydrate 12 g · Fiber 5 g · Fat 10 g · Saturated Fat 1 g · Sodium 216

Rye Rolls with Chocolate

MAKES 12

If you are fond of *pain au chocolate*, you will enjoy this earthier version made with whole wheat flour and crunchy sunflower seeds. They freeze well, so you can defrost one when you need a bit of something sweet.

2 cups water

½ cup low-fat plain skyr or Cheater's Skyr (page 231)

½ teaspoon instant yeast

2 cups whole wheat flour

1 cup unbleached all-purpose flour, plus more for dusting

1 cup rye flour

2 teaspoons salt

2 ounces bittersweet chocolate (about 70% cacao), coarsely chopped

⅓ cup raw sunflower seeds

Vegetable oil, for greasing the baking sheet

Mix the water, skyr, and yeast in a large bowl. Add the whole wheat, unbleached, and rye flours and the salt and stir until just combined. Add the chocolate and sunflower seeds and knead in the bowl for 6 to 7 minutes to make a somewhat tacky dough. Do not add too much flour. Cover the bowl with a damp kitchen towel and let rise until doubled, about 1 hour.

Turn the dough out onto a lightly floured work surface and roll it into a 24-inch log. Using a sharp knife, cut the dough crosswise on an angle into 12 equal triangles. Lightly grease a large baking sheet and place the triangles of dough on it, leaving a little space between each. Cover with a damp kitchen towel and set aside in a warm, draft-free place until the rolls look puffy, about 30 minutes.

Preheat the oven to 425°F.

Bake the rolls for 20 minutes, or until they sound hollow when tapped on the base. Serve warm or at room temperature.

To store, wrap each roll well in plastic wrap and freeze for up to 2 months. Thaw as needed.

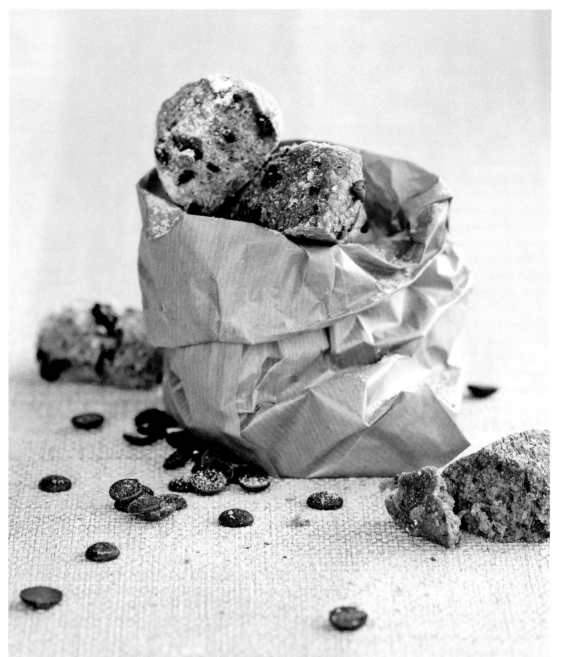

RATIO (Carb:Protein) = 4:1

PER SERVING: Calories 200 • Protein 7 g • Carbohydrate 31 g • Fiber 5 g • Fat 4 g •
Saturated Fat 1 g • Sodium 387 mg

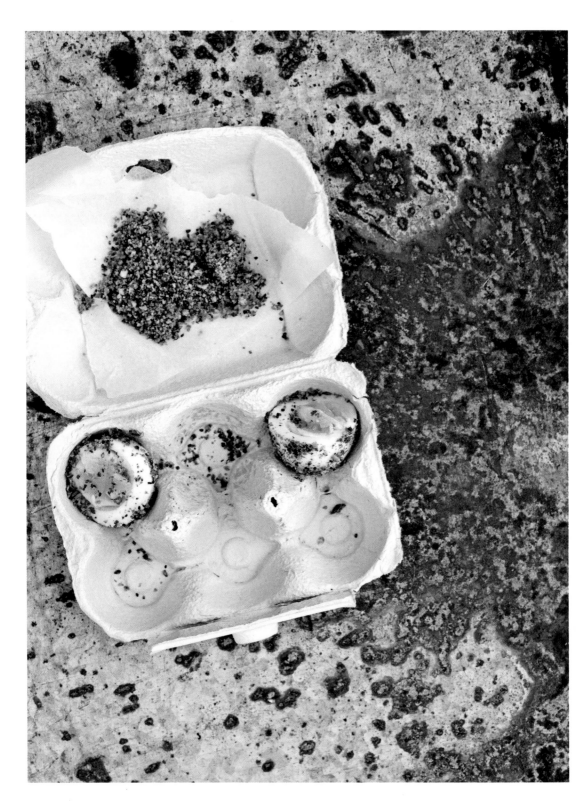

Crunchy Egg

SERVES 1

This snack is practically pure protein, a good way to balance an otherwise carb-heavy meal.

1 teaspoon finely chopped raw almonds

1 teaspoon skinned hazelnuts

1 teaspoon raw unsalted hulled pumpkin seeds (pepitas)

1 teaspoon hulled sunflower seeds

Salt

1 large egg, hard-boiled

Toast the almonds, hazelnuts, pumpkin seeds, and sunflower seeds in a skillet over medium heat, stirring often, until lightly browned, 3 to 5 minutes. Finely chop the nuts and seeds by hand or transfer to a small food processor and pulse to chop, then add a little salt and mix to combine. Peel the egg, cut it in half, and roll it in the toasted nut-seed mixture.

RATIO (Carb:Protein) = 1:8

PER SERVING: Calories 130 • Protein 8 g • Carbohydrate 1 g • Fiber 1 g • Fat 10 g • Saturated Fat 2 g • Sodium 173 mg

Carrots with Green Pea Dip

SERVES 2

Add this to your party rotation; its bright green color makes it a festive alternative to the more expected hummus. Or divide the dip between two containers for two pack-along afternoon snacks.

2¼ cups frozen peas

2 tablespoons toasted unsalted hulled pumpkin seeds (pepitas)

Juice of ½ lemon

1 tablespoon canola oil

1 teaspoon ground cumin

1 garlic clove, finely chopped

Salt and freshly ground black pepper

4 carrots, halved lengthwise

Cook the peas in a saucepan of salted boiling water for 4 to 5 minutes, until tender. Drain the water, reserving some in case you need to adjust the texture later.

Transfer the peas to a food processor or blender, add the pumpkin seeds, lemon juice, oil, cumin, and garlic, and process to combine. Season with salt and pepper. Add a little of the reserved cooking water if the mixture is too thick.

Serve the green pea dip with the carrots.

RATIO (Carb:Protein) = 1:1

PER SERVING: Calories 250 · Protein 10 g · Carbohydrate 12 g · Fiber 11 g · Fat 16 g · Saturated Fat 2 g · Sodium 111 mg

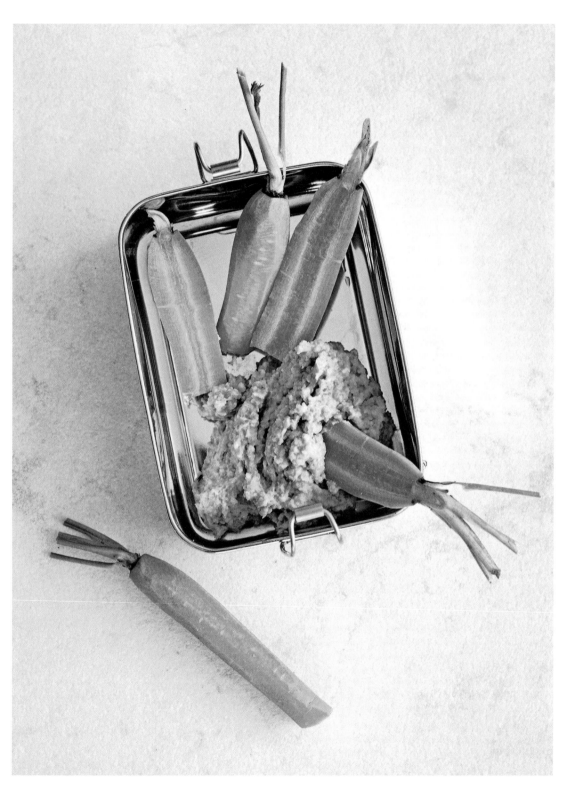

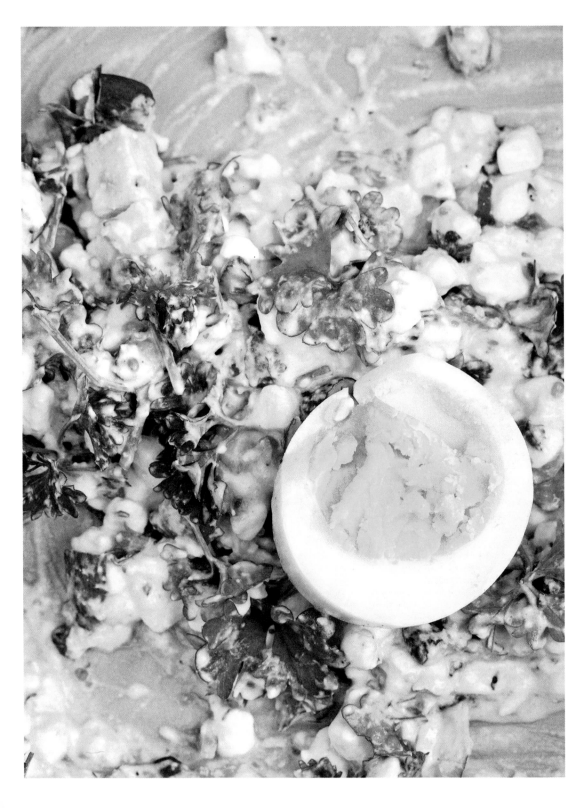

Egg with
Cottage Cheese & Almonds

SERVES 1

Don't omit the parsley from this simple-to-assemble snack; it adds color and a fresh herbaceous note.

2 tablespoons cottage cheese

2 tablespoons chopped toasted raw almonds (see Note)

Handful of fresh parsley leaves

1 teaspoon Dijon mustard

1 large egg, hard-boiled and cut in half

Mix the cottage cheese, almonds, parsley, and mustard in a small bowl. Place on a plate or in a bowl and serve with the egg.

NOTE: To toast almonds, preheat the oven to 350°F. Spread the almonds on a baking sheet and bake, stirring occasionally, until they look and smell toasted, about 10 minutes. Let cool before chopping.

RATIO (Carb:Protein) = 1:6

PER SERVING: Calories 255 · Protein 17 g · Carbohydrate 3 g · Fiber 4 g · Fat 19 g · Saturated Fat 4 g · Sodium 219 mg

Pita with Cottage Cheese & Apple

SERVES 1

If you have dismissed cottage cheese as old-school diet food, give it another look. With far fewer calories than ricotta cheese, it's a creamy, satisfying protein source that complements many other flavors. Be sure to choose low-fat over "creamed" full-fat varieties.

2 tablespoons cottage cheese

1 apple, cored and diced

1 tablespoon sesame seeds, toasted (see Note)

½ low-GI whole-grain pita bread, cut into triangles and toasted

Mix the cottage cheese, apple, and sesame seeds in a small bowl. Serve the pita triangles topped with the cottage cheese mixture.

NOTE: To toast sesame seeds, heat a small skillet over medium heat. Add the seeds and toast, stirring occasionally, until they are beginning to brown, 1 to 2 minutes. Immediately transfer to a plate and let cool.

RATIO (Carb:Protein) = 3:1

PER SERVING: Calories 419 · Protein 17 g · Carbohydrate 51 g · Fiber 9 g · Fat 15 g · Saturated Fat 3 g · Sodium 433 mg

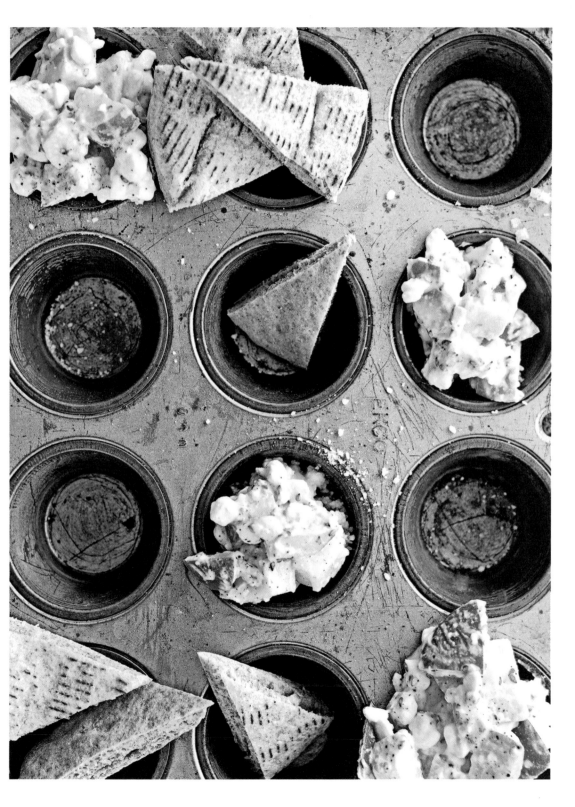

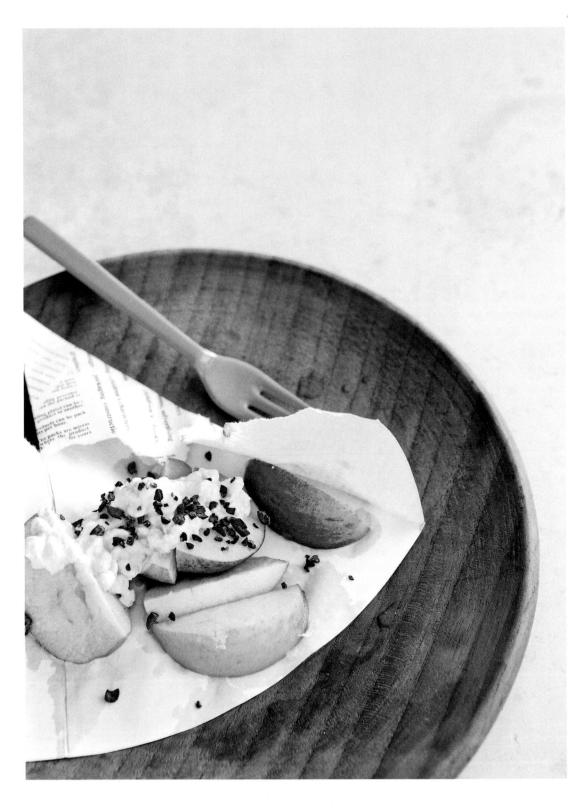

Apple with
Lemon & Cocoa Nibs

SERVES 1

Cocoa nibs are packed with antioxidants and deliver a powerful chocolate punch without sweetness.

1 apple or pear, cored and cut into thin wedges

Juice of ½ lemon

Scant ½ cup cottage cheese

1 tablespoon cocoa nibs

Sprinkle the apple with the lemon juice. Serve with the cottage cheese and cocoa nibs.

RATIO (Carb:Protein) = 2:1

PER SERVING: Calories 324 · Protein 19 g · Carbohydrate 27 g · Fiber 3 g · Fat 15 g · Saturated Fat 9 g · Sodium 283 mg

Pear with
Pepper & Mozzarella

SERVES 1

A perfect example of everyday ingredients combined in a way that is at once simple and elegant.

1 pear, cored and cut into wedges

2 ounces fresh mozzarella, cut into bite-size pieces

1 teaspoon honey

Freshly ground black pepper

Serve the pear wedges and mozzarella drizzled with the honey and lightly topped with pepper.

RATIO (Carb:Protein) = 2:1

PER SERVING: Calories 275 · Protein 14 g · Carbohydrate 29 g · Fiber 4 g · Fat 11 g · Saturated Fat 7 g · Sodium 234 mg

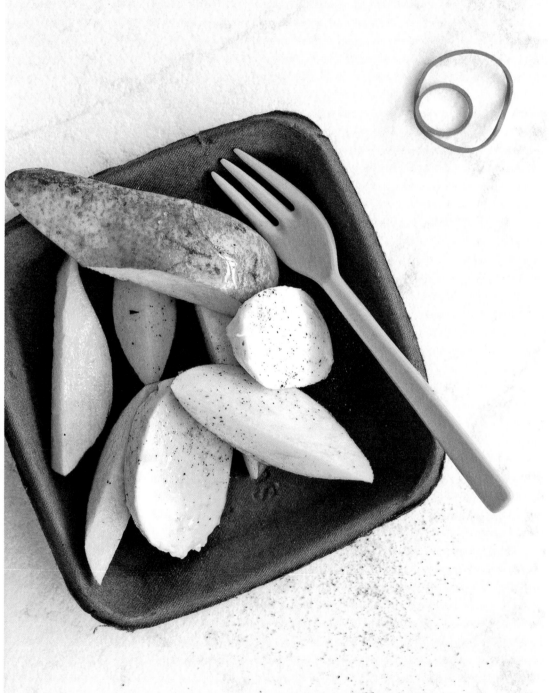

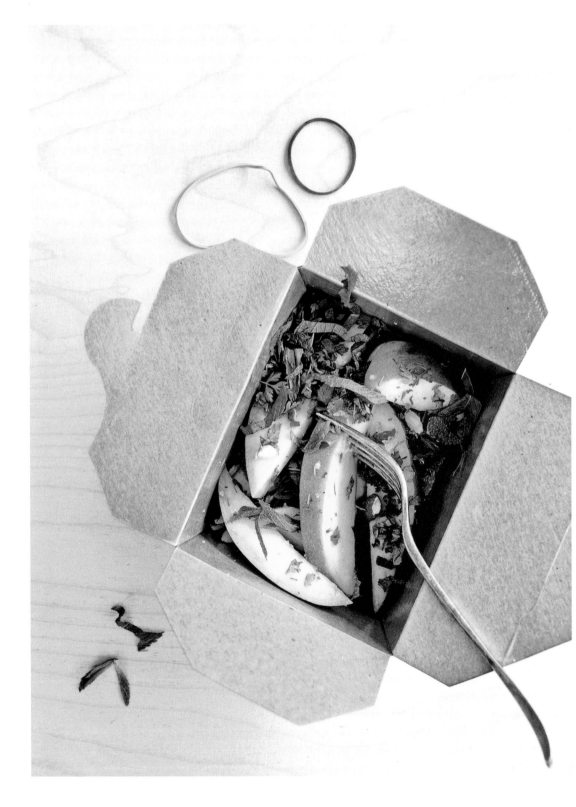

Mango, Almonds & Mint

So flavorful, so sophisticated, and so easy. Be sure to use a ripe, fragrant mango for the best flavor.

½ mango, peeled and cut into wedges

½ apple, cored and cut into wedges

Coarsely chopped fresh mint or chervil leaves

10 whole raw almonds, toasted and chopped (see page 99)

½ teaspoon salt

¼ cup low-fat plain skyr or Cheater's Skyr (page 231), for serving

Serve the mango and apple sprinkled with the mint, almonds, and a little salt, with the skyr alongside.

RATIO (Carb:Protein) = 5:1

PER SERVING: Calories 165 · Protein 4 g · Carbohydrate 20 g · Fiber 5 g · Fat 7 g · Saturated Fat <1 g · Sodium 605 mg

Crispy Kiwifruit

High-fiber kiwi gets a protein boost here from a coating of nuts and seeds.

1 tablespoon finely chopped
toasted raw almonds (see
page 99)

1 teaspoon toasted unsalted
hulled pumpkin seeds
(pepitas)

Freshly ground black pepper

1 kiwifruit, peeled and cut into
wedges

Mix together the almonds, pepitas, and a little pepper in a small bowl. Serve the kiwi wedges dipped in the almond mixture.

RATIO (Carb:Protein) = 3:2

PER SERVING: Calories 170 · Protein 6 g · Carbohydrate 9 g · Fiber 5 g · Fat 11 g · Saturated Fat 1 g · Sodium 6 mg

Chilled Tomato Soup

SERVES 2

A refreshing variation on gazpacho.

1 (14.5-ounce) can diced tomatoes

1 ripe fresh tomato, chopped

½ green bell pepper, seeded and finely chopped

¼ seedless (English) cucumber, diced

1 teaspoon chili powder

Handful of fresh basil leaves, torn

1 garlic clove, minced

2 drops of hot sauce

1 teaspoon olive oil

Salt and freshly ground black pepper

2 lean bacon slices, cooked and crumbled

Combine the canned tomatoes with their juice, the fresh tomato, bell pepper, cucumber, lime juice, chili powder, basil, garlic, hot sauce, and olive oil in a blender and process until combined and smooth with just a little texture. Season with salt and black pepper. Refrigerate in an airtight container for at least 4 hours, but preferably overnight so the flavors can develop.

For each serving, spoon half the soup into an individual soup bowl and top with half the crumbled bacon. Serve chilled.

RATIO (Carb:Protein) = 3:1

PER SERVING: Calories 95 · Protein 3 g · Carbohydrate 10 g · Fiber 5 g · Fat 3 g · Saturated Fat <1 g · Sodium 230 mg

Quinoa with Roast Beef, Tomato & Watercress

Bowl cuisine is here to stay; this combo is homey yet full of bright flavors.

¼ cup quinoa, rinsed and drained

4 ounces deli-sliced rare roast beef, cut into strips

2 small radishes, thinly sliced

4 cherry tomatoes, halved

1 cup watercress, thick stems discarded

About 10 fresh mint leaves

2 teaspoons fresh lemon juice

1 teaspoon olive oil

Salt and freshly ground black pepper

Mix the quinoa and ½ cup water in a small saucepan. Bring to a boil over medium heat. Reduce the heat to low and cover. Simmer for 12 minutes, or until the water has been absorbed. Remove from the heat and cool completely.

Put the quinoa, roast beef, radish, tomato, watercress, and mint in a bowl or on a plate. Dress with the lemon juice and olive oil, and season with salt and pepper.

RATIO (Carb:Protein) = 1:2

PER SERVING: Calories 254 · Protein 25 g · Carbohydrate 17 g · Fiber 6 g · Fat 9 g · Saturated Fat 2 g · Sodium 1,212 mg

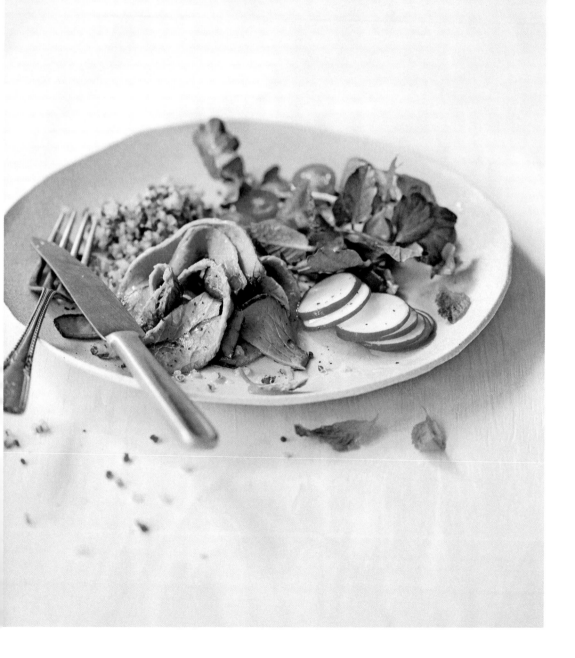

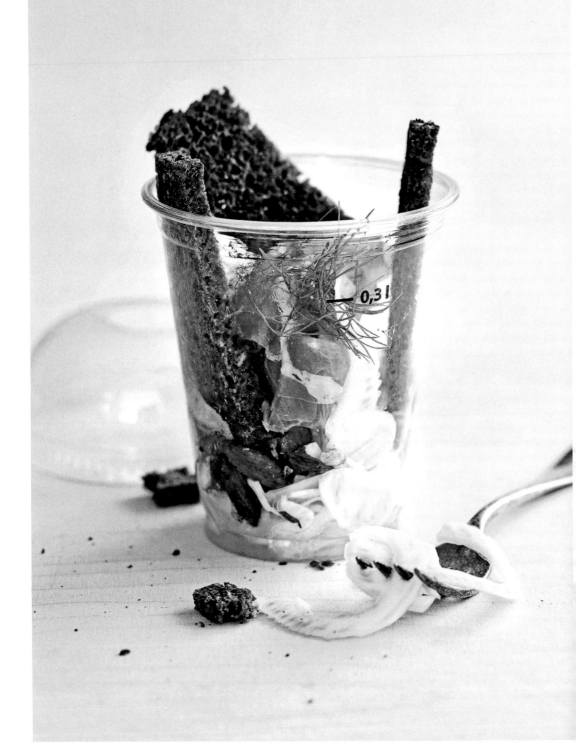

Fennel, Prosciutto & Almonds

All your senses will be engaged by this alluring blend of sweet, salty, crunchy, and tangy ingredients.

½ fennel bulb

1 tablespoon chopped raw
    almonds

Zest and juice of ½ lemon

Honey

Salt and freshly ground black
    pepper

2 slices prosciutto

½ slice whole-grain rye bread
    or whole rye pumpernickel
    bread, toasted and cut into
    strips

1 sprig fresh dill

Remove the tough outer layer of the fennel and discard. Using a mandoline or a sharp knife, thinly slice the bulb crosswise horizontally. Put the fennel in a medium bowl and mix in the almonds, lemon zest, lemon juice, and honey. Season with salt and pepper. Add the prosciutto and toasted bread, garnish with the dill, and serve.

RATIO (Carb:Protein) = 3:1

PER SERVING: Calories 337 · Protein 16 g · Carbohydrate 45 g · Fiber 5 g · Fat 9 g · Saturated Fat 1 g · Sodium 1,055 mg

Rye Berries with Cucumber & Hazelnuts

SERVES 1

Though not traditionally Scandinavian, fish sauce adds a note of umami savoriness to dishes that makes them especially satisfying.

Salt

⅓ cup rye berries or pearled barley

¼ seedless (English) cucumber, cut into bite-size pieces

1 ounce Parmesan cheese, diced

1 tablespoon coarsely chopped skinned toasted hazelnuts (see page 80)

Small handful of fresh basil leaves

1 tablespoon apple cider vinegar

1 teaspoon Thai fish sauce

Dash of canola oil

Freshly ground black pepper

Bring a medium saucepan of salted water to a boil over high heat. Add the rye and reduce the heat to medium. Cook the rye until it is tender, 20 to 30 minutes. Drain in a sieve, rinse under cold running water, and let cool.

Combine the rye, cucumber, cheese, hazelnuts, and basil in a medium bowl. Whisk the vinegar, fish sauce, and oil together in a small bowl. Add to the salad and toss to combine. Season with salt and pepper.

RATIO (Carb:Protein) = 1:1

PER SERVING: Calories 310 • Protein 12 g • Carbohydrate 12 g • Fiber 4 g • Fat 23 g • Saturated Fat 8 g • Sodium 847 mg

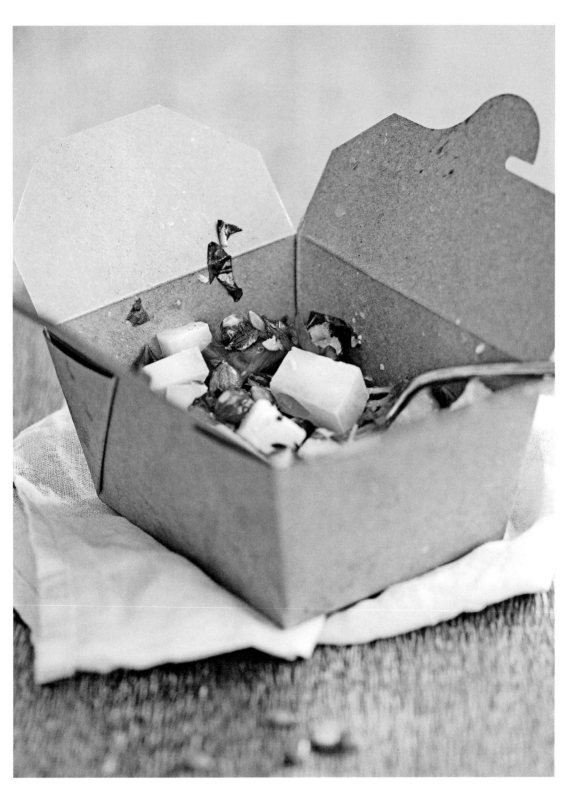

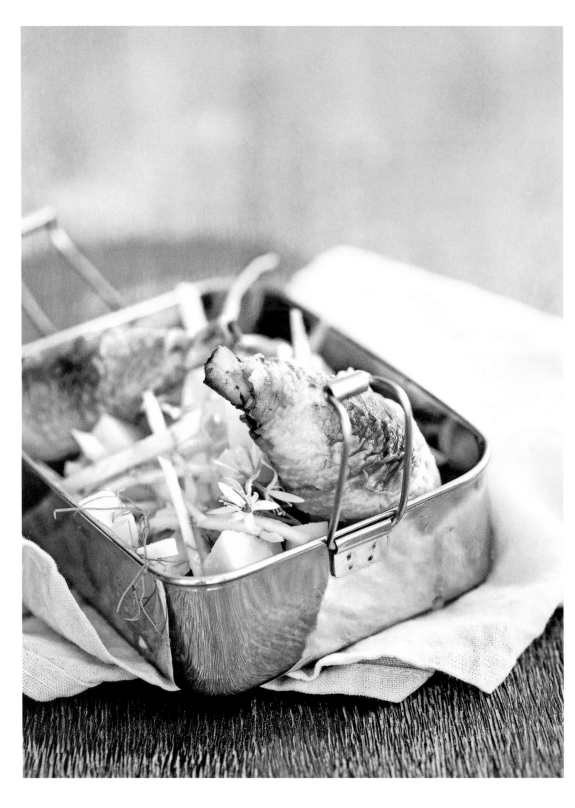

Chicken Salad

If you have leftover cooked pork loin, turkey, or roast beef, they can readily be substituted for the chicken in this versatile salad. It keeps well, so don't hesitate to double the recipe.

½ green, savoy, or napa cabbage, thinly shredded

½ cup diced Emmental cheese

Handful of fresh dill fronds

2 tablespoons Dijon mustard

Juice of 1 lemon

2 tablespoons honey

2 tablespoons canola oil

Salt and freshly ground black pepper

8 ounces cooked skinless chicken meat

Combine the cabbage, cheese, and dill in a salad bowl. Whisk together the mustard, lemon juice, honey, and oil in a small bowl. Add to the salad and toss to combine. Season with salt and pepper. Serve the salad topped with the chicken.

RATIO (Carb:Protein) = 1:1

PER SERVING: Calories 577 · Protein 39 g · Carbohydrate 35 g · Fiber 7 g · Fat 31 g · Saturated Fat 7 g · Sodium 802 mg

Soba Noodles with Tofu, Ginger & Sugar Snaps

A serious improvement over packaged noodles, this veggie-rich version has a fraction of the sodium and far more beneficial nutrients.

1½ ounces dried soba noodles

1 cup sugar snap peas, trimmed and sliced

3 ounces marinated baked tofu, thinly sliced

¼ red bell pepper, seeded and thinly sliced

1 cup packed Asian-blend salad greens or baby spinach

2 teaspoons reduced-sodium soy sauce

1 teaspoon mirin

½ teaspoon finely grated fresh ginger

Bring a medium saucepan of water to a boil over high heat. Add the soba noodles and cook according to the package directions until al dente. During the last 30 seconds, add the sugar snap peas. Drain the noodles and peas in a colander and rinse well under cold running water.

Combine the noodles, sugar snap peas, tofu, bell pepper, and salad leaves in an individual salad bowl. Add the soy sauce, mirin, and ginger, toss gently, and serve.

RATIO (Carb:Protein) = 1:1

PER SERVING: Calories 198 · Protein 16 g · Carbohydrate 12 g · Fiber 11 g · Fat 7 g · Saturated Fat 1 g · Sodium 399 mg

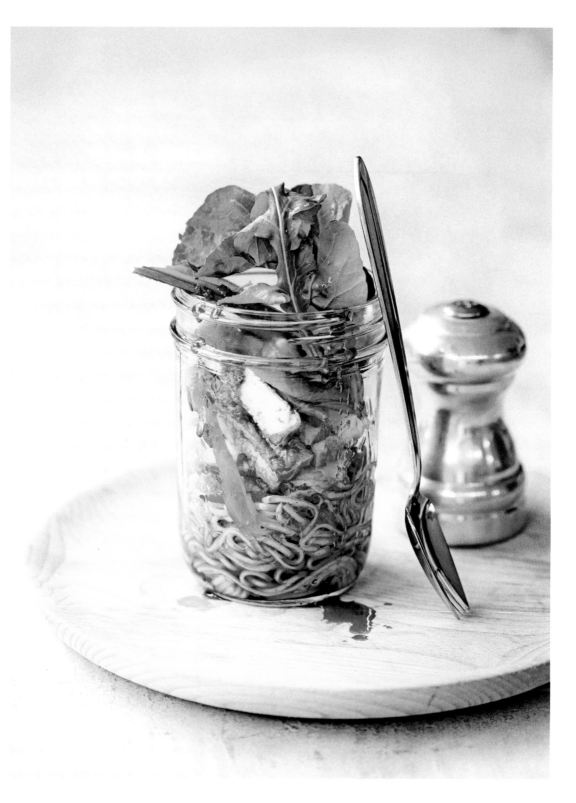

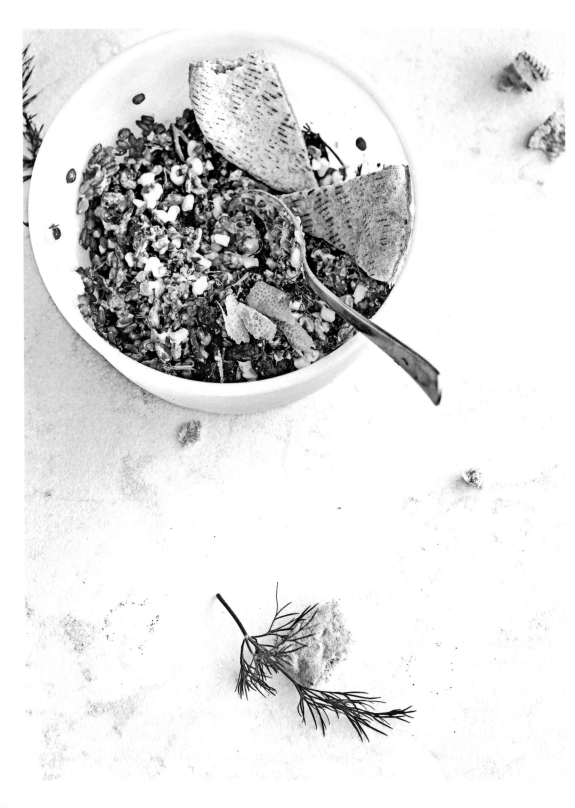

Rye Salad with Lemon & Berries

Another way to use rye, this time as the basis of a chewy, substantial salad. Serve with pita bread, if desired (note, bread not included in analysis below).

Salt

⅓ cup rye berries or pearled barley

½ cup cottage cheese

Handful of fresh herbs

Zest and juice of 1 lemon

1 tablespoon canola oil

1 tablespoon fresh or thawed frozen berries

½ low-GI whole wheat pita bread, for serving (optional)

Bring a medium saucepan of salted water to a boil over high heat. Add the rye and reduce the heat to medium. Cook the rye until it is tender, 20 to 30 minutes. Drain in a sieve, rinse under cold running water, and let cool.

Put the rye, cottage cheese, herbs, lemon zest, lemon juice, oil, and berries in an individual salad bowl and gently toss to combine.

RATIO (Carb:Protein) = 2:1

PER SERVING: Calories 483 • Protein 21 g • Carbohydrate 37 g • Fiber 2 g • Fat 26 g • Saturated Fat 5 g • Sodium 296 mg

Tuna, Potatoes & Eggs

SERVES 2

Sour, bitter, and tangy elements reinvent tuna salad for a dish that is anything but bland.

1 (5-ounce) can tuna packed in water, drained

2 bitter lettuce leaves, such as radicchio or escarole

4 small fingerling potatoes, boiled and sliced

2 small sour pickles, sliced

2 tablespoons fresh lemon juice

1 tablespoon olive oil

Salt and freshly ground black pepper

1 large egg, hard-boiled and cut in half

Combine the tuna, lettuce, potatoes, and pickles in a medium bowl. Whisk together the lemon juice and olive oil in a small bowl, add to the salad, and gently toss to combine. Season with salt and pepper, and serve with the hard-boiled egg.

RATIO (Carb:Protein) = 1:1

PER SERVING: Calories 393 · Protein 30 g · Carbohydrate 34 g · Fiber 4 g · Fat 14 g · Saturated Fat 3 g · Sodium 530 mg

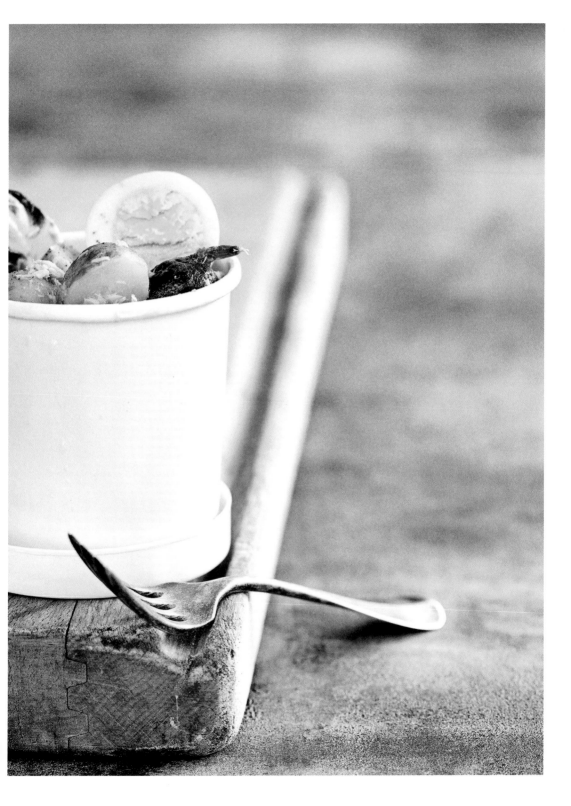

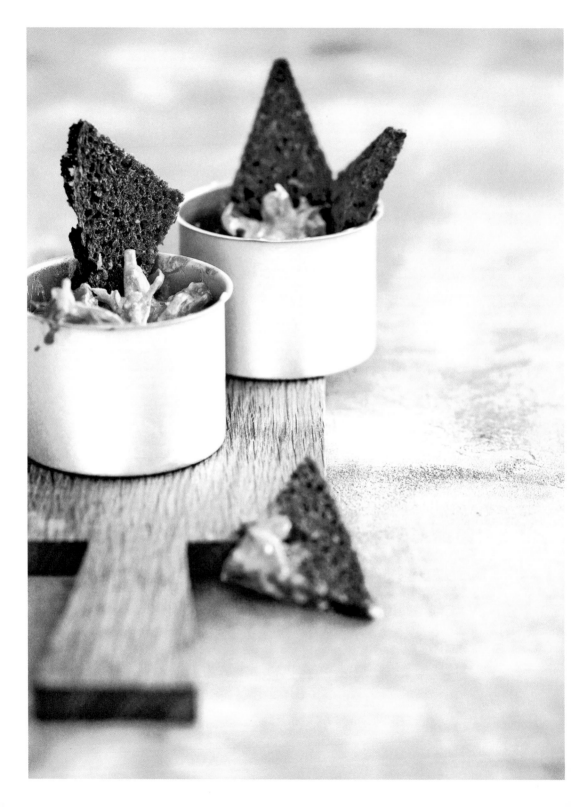

Mackerel, Cabbage & Rye Bread

SERVES 1

Mackerel is little used in North America but it is an inexpensive, sustainable protein source that is convenient to keep on hand—qualities that should move it to the top of your shopping list.

2 tablespoons low-fat plain skyr or Cheater's Skyr (page 231)

1 teaspoon Dijon mustard

¼ head green, savoy, or napa cabbage, very thinly sliced

1 (4.25-ounce) can mackerel or sardines in tomato sauce

1 tablespoon coarsely chopped toasted raw almonds (see page 99)

Small handful of fresh dill leaves

Salt and freshly ground black pepper

1 slice whole-grain rye bread or whole rye pumpernickel bread, toasted

Mix the skyr and mustard together in an individual salad bowl until well combined. Gently mix in the cabbage, mackerel, almonds, dill, and salt and pepper to taste.

Serve with the toasted bread.

RATIO (Carb:Protein) = 1:1

PER SERVING: Calories 476 · Protein 39 g · Carbohydrate 31 g · Fiber 10 g · Fat 20 g · Saturated Fat 4 g · Sodium 932 mg

Chicken, Corn & Cornichons

Throw an extra chicken breast or two on the grill next time you barbecue so you'll have cooked chicken on hand for this summertime salad. It doubles easily.

1 small ear corn, husked

3½ ounces cooked chicken, shredded (about 1 cup loosely packed)

1 tablespoon pitted black olives

3 cornichons, sliced

1 small tomato, halved

1 tablespoon olive oil

Salt and freshly ground black pepper

Bring a medium saucepan of water to a boil over high heat. Add the corn and boil for 5 to 10 minutes, until tender. Drain, rinse under cold running water, and let cool. Stand the corn on its wide end and slice the kernels from the cob.

In an individual salad bowl, combine the corn, chicken, olives, cornichons, tomato, and olive oil and mix. Season with salt and pepper.

RATIO (Carb:Protein) = 3:4

PER SERVING: Calories 493 · Protein 32 g · Carbohydrate 24 g · Fiber 8 g · Fat 28 g · Saturated Fat 4 g · Sodium 671 mg

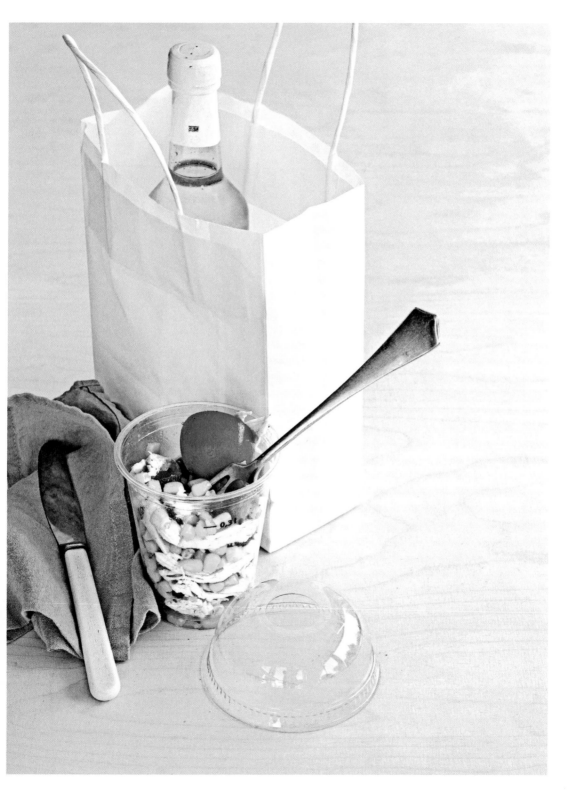

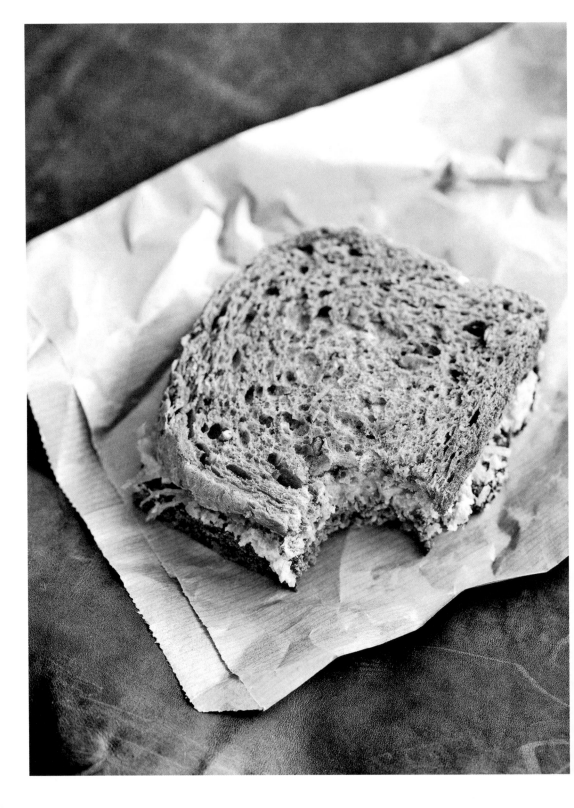

Two-Bread Sandwich

SERVES 1

Though it may seem strange at first blush, swapping out one of your wheat bread slices for rye makes any sandwich more GI-friendly.

1 slice whole-grain rye bread or whole rye pumpernickel bread

1 tablespoon Dijon mustard

3 tablespoons Hummus (page 206)

1 slice lean cooked ham, fat trimmed

1 carrot, shredded

1 slice low-GI whole wheat bread

Spread the mustard on the rye bread. Top with the hummus, followed by the ham and carrot. Add the whole wheat bread and serve.

RATIO (Carb:Protein) = 4:1

PER SERVING: Calories 373 · Protein 12 g · Carbohydrate 41 g · Fiber 11 g · Fat 16 g · Saturated Fat 1 g · Sodium 848 mg

Beggar's Purses with Hummus & Cottage Cheese

SERVES 1

Another unexpected use for hummus, here as the protein-rich filling for little baked dumplings. Chia seeds add still more protein, as well as a bit of visual interest.

3 teaspoons Hummus
(page 206)

6 wonton wrappers

1 large egg, whisked

2 tablespoons chia seeds

3 teaspoons cottage cheese

Preheat the oven to 400°F. Line a baking sheet with parchment paper.

Place 1 teaspoon of the hummus in the center of a wonton wrapper and gather up the edges to make a pouch. Brush the edges with the whisked egg and sprinkle with some of the chia seeds. Place on the baking sheet. Repeat to make two more hummus-filled dumplings, then repeat with the remaining wontons and the cottage cheese.

Bake the wontons for 10 minutes, or until browned and crisp.

RATIO (Carb:Protein) = 2:1

PER SERVING: Calories 396 · Protein 18 g · Carbohydrate 31 g · Fiber 8 g · Fat 20 g · Saturated Fat 3 g · Sodium 264 mg

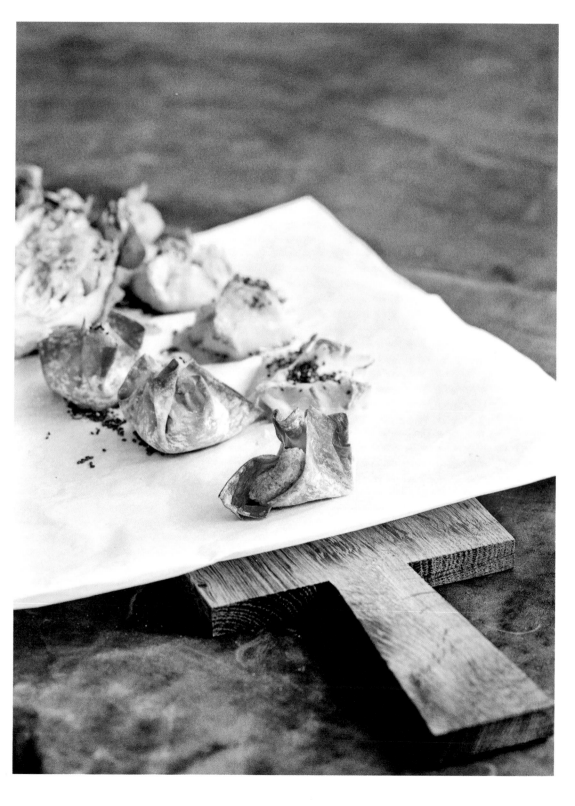

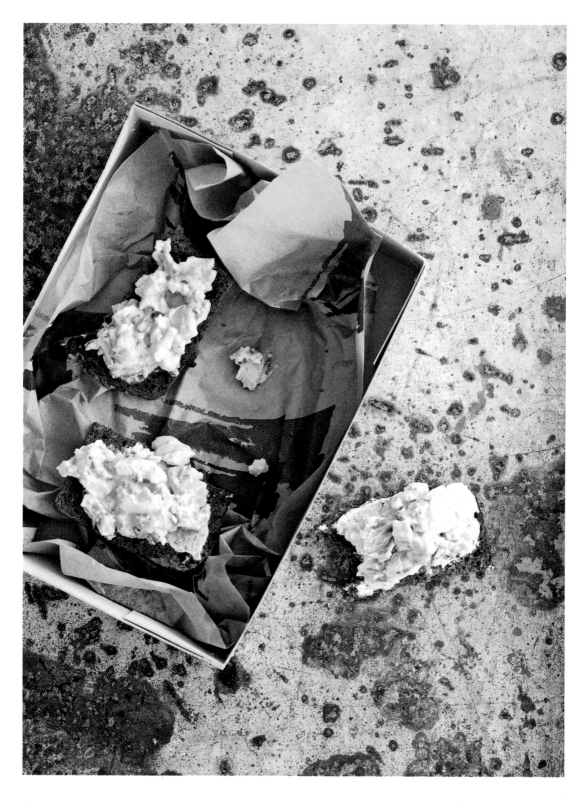

Egg & Vegetable Salad
on Toasted Rye

SERVES 1

Egg salad on rye is a classic pairing that gets a big flavor boost from curry powder and lots of crisp vegetables. Serve it open-faced if you want to further reduce the carb ratio.

½ cup low-fat plain skyr or Cheater's Skyr (page 231)

1 teaspoon curry powder

¼ seedless (English) cucumber, chopped

½ small green bell pepper, seeded and chopped

2 cauliflower florets, chopped

½ small red onion, finely chopped

1 small sour dill pickle, diced

2 large eggs, hard-boiled and diced

Salt and freshly ground black pepper

2 slices whole-grain rye bread or whole rye pumpernickel bread, toasted

Mix the skyr and curry powder together in a bowl until combined. Mix in the cucumber, bell pepper, cauliflower florets, red onion, and pickle. Fold in the hard-boiled eggs and season with salt and black pepper.

Serve the egg salad spooned over the toasted bread.

RATIO (Carb:Protein) = 5:3

PER SERVING: Calories 471 · Protein 36 g · Carbohydrate 54 g · Fiber 9 g · Fat 10 g · Saturated Fat 3 g · Sodium 691 mg

Stuffed Peppers with Lamb, Quinoa & Lemon

SERVES 1

Preserved lemon is used widely in Middle Eastern cuisines, especially that of Morocco. They are an easy way to add a citrusy complexity to grain dishes, stews, and other recipes and offer a counterpoint here to the sweet currants and meaty lamb.

⅓ cup quinoa, rinsed and drained

2½ ounces lean ground lamb

½ zucchini, trimmed and shredded

1 tablespoon rinsed and finely chopped Moroccan-style preserved lemon (remove white pith before chopping)

1 tablespoon chopped fresh parsley

2 teaspoons dried currants

¼ teaspoon red pepper flakes

Salt and freshly ground black pepper

1 large red bell pepper, halved and seeded

1½ cups mixed salad greens, for serving

Combine the quinoa and ⅔ cup water in a small saucepan and bring to a boil over medium heat. Reduce the heat to low, cover, and simmer for about 12 minutes, or until the water has been absorbed. Remove from the heat and let cool.

Preheat the oven to 350°F. Line a baking sheet with parchment paper.

Mix the quinoa, lamb, zucchini, preserved lemon, parsley, currants, and red pepper flakes in a medium bowl. Season with salt and black pepper.

Spoon the quinoa mixture into the bell pepper halves and place them on the baking sheet or in an ovenproof skillet. Cover with aluminum foil. Bake for 20 minutes. Remove the foil and bake for 10 to 15 minutes more, or until the peppers are tender. Serve with the salad leaves alongside.

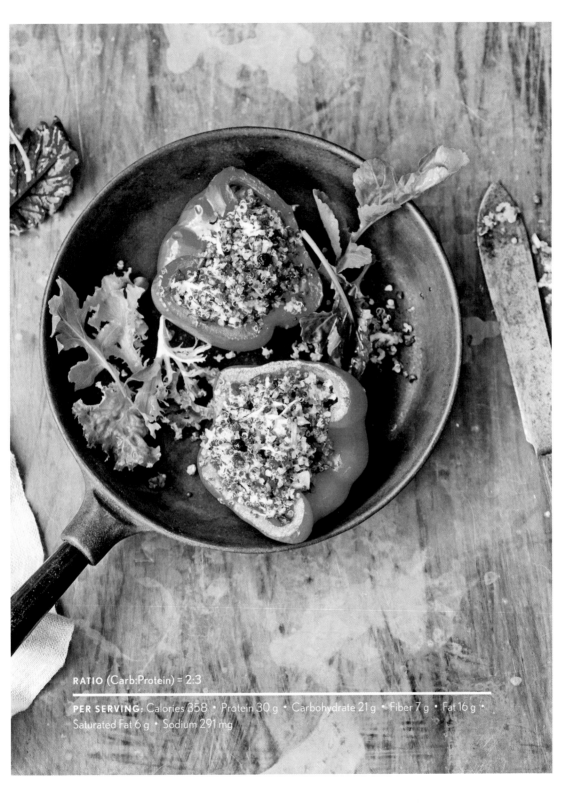

RATIO (Carb:Protein) = 2:3

PER SERVING: Calories 358 • Protein 30 g • Carbohydrate 21 g • Fiber 7 g • Fat 16 g • Saturated Fat 6 g • Sodium 291 mg

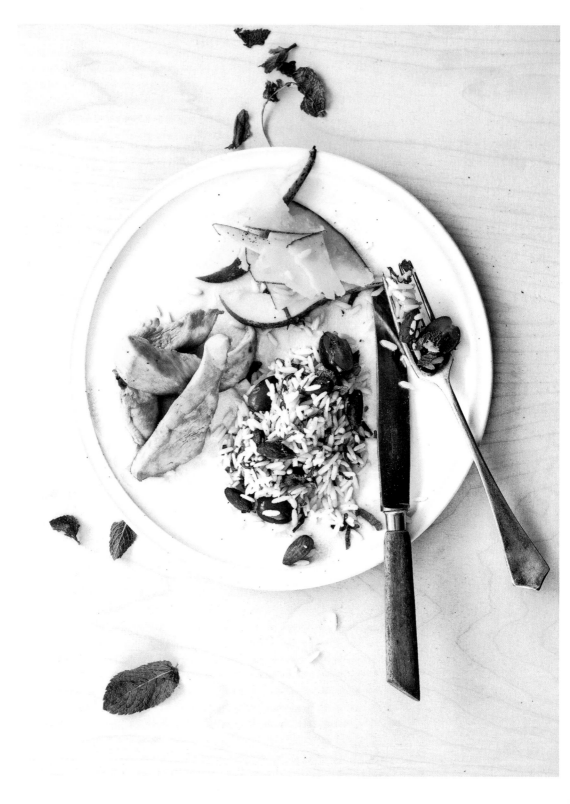

Chicken Breast with Pears, Grapes & Rice

SERVES 1

A simple supper with a satisfying blend of flavors, textures, and colors. You may need to search out lower-GI rice online, but it's worth the effort.

¼ cup low-GI basmati rice, such as Laxmi

Olive oil spray

3 ounces boneless, skinless chicken breast

1 pear, cut into wedges

1 tablespoon honey

1 ounce Pecorino Romano cheese, very thinly sliced

Salt and freshly ground black pepper

10 purple grapes, halved

Small handful of fresh mint leaves, shredded

1 tablespoon chopped raw almonds

Bring a small saucepan of water to a boil over high heat. Add the rice and reduce the heat to medium-low. Simmer until the rice is tender, about 20 minutes, or according to package directions.

Meanwhile, coat a nonstick skillet with olive oil spray. Add the chicken and cook over medium heat, turning once, for about 8 minutes, or until just cooked through.

Mix the pear wedges, honey, and cheese in a small bowl. Season with salt and pepper.

Drain the rice and transfer to a small bowl. Mix in the grapes, mint, and almonds, and season with salt and pepper.

Slice the chicken and serve with the rice mixture and the pear salad.

RATIO (Carb:Protein) = 3:2

PER SERVING: Calories 647 · Protein 54 g · Carbohydrate 83 g · Fiber 5 g · Fat 12 g · Saturated Fat 2 g · Sodium 533 mg

Meatballs with Edamame & Cabbage

SERVES 4

While Swedish meatballs get all the press, our leaner, lower-GI version is every bit as tasty and much better for you. Honey adds a subtle sweetness; you'll never miss the lingonberry sauce.

9 ounces ground veal

9 ounces lean ground beef

⅔ cup rolled rye flakes or rolled oats, plus more if needed

3 large eggs, beaten

6 tablespoons milk

6 tablespoons apple juice

1 garlic clove, finely chopped

Salt and freshly ground black pepper

2 tablespoons canola oil

½ cup cottage cheese

1 tablespoon honey

Juice of ½ lemon

¼ green cabbage, cored and finely shredded

¼ cup frozen shelled edamame, thawed

Coarsely chopped fresh dill

Put the ground veal, ground beef, rye flakes, eggs, milk, apple juice, and garlic in a bowl. Season with a little salt and pepper and use your hands to mix until well combined. If the mixture is too wet, add some more rye flakes. You should be able to shape the mixture into 16 meatballs that will hold their shape.

Heat the oil in a nonstick skillet over medium-high heat. Add the meatballs and cook, turning often, until browned all over and cooked through, about 10 minutes. (Alternatively, you can sear them in the skillet, then transfer to a parchment paper–lined baking sheet and bake in a preheated 325°F oven to finish cooking if you prefer—they should need 5 to 8 minutes in the oven.)

Mix together the cottage cheese, honey, and lemon juice in a small bowl. Season with salt and pepper.

Mix the cabbage, edamame, and dill in a medium bowl.

Serve the meatballs with the cabbage and cottage cheese mixtures.

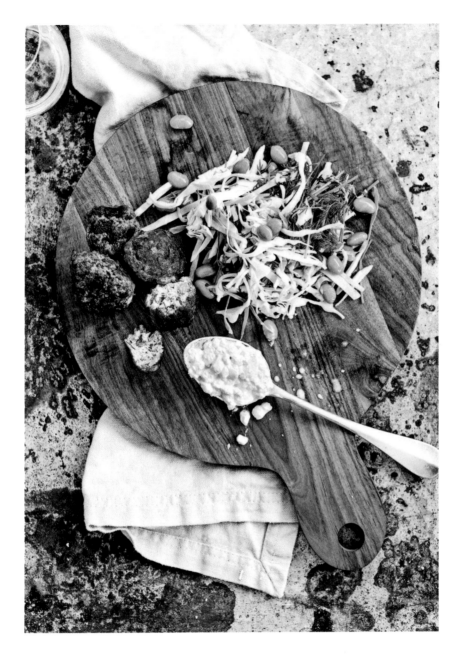

RATIO (Carb:Protein) = 3:5

PER SERVING: Calories 513 · Protein 53 g · Carbohydrate 31 g · Fiber 3 g · Fat 19 g · Saturated Fat 4 g · Sodium 265 mg

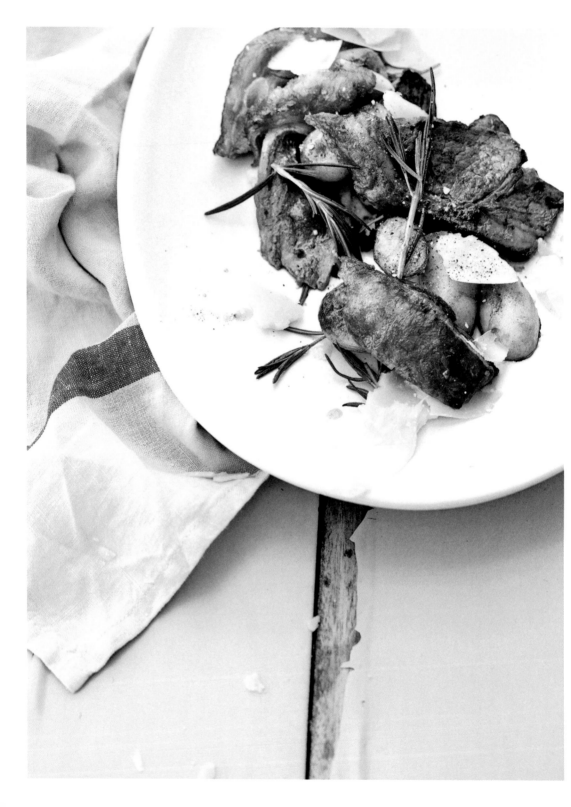

Beef with
Salt & Vinegar Potatoes

SERVES 1

A healthier take on steak frites (or salt-and-vinegar potato chips!). Be sure to round out the meal with plenty of vegetables.

Olive oil spray

5 ounces beef tenderloin

4 small or 2 medium fingerling potatoes, peeled and cut into thin bite-size pieces

3½ tablespoons apple cider vinegar

6 tablespoons water

1 fresh rosemary sprig, plus more for serving

Salt and freshly ground black pepper

Shaved Parmesan cheese, for serving

Coat a nonstick skillet or ridged grill pan with olive oil spray and heat over medium-high heat. Add the steak and cook for 2 to 3 minutes on each side. Transfer to a cutting board and let rest while you cook the potatoes.

Return the skillet to medium heat. Add the potatoes and cook, turning often, until lightly browned, about 5 minutes. Add the vinegar, water, rosemary, and some salt. Bring to a boil and cook, without stirring, until the liquid has evaporated and the potatoes are tender with a light crust forming on one side, about 4 minutes more. Give the pan a good shake to release the potatoes. Season with pepper.

Slice the steak and transfer to a plate. Add the potatoes, scatter with the cheese and rosemary, and serve.

RATIO (Carb:Protein) = 1:1

PER SERVING: Calories 552 · Protein 43 g · Carbohydrate 36 g · Fiber 5 g · Fat 24 g · Saturated Fat 10 g · Sodium 375 mg

Salmon with Avocado, Peas & Fennel

Salmon is a dinner table fixture throughout Scandinavia. Choose wild-caught when possible, organically farmed otherwise.

5 ounces salmon fillet

1 teaspoon ground cumin

½ cup frozen peas

1 avocado, pitted, peeled, and finely diced

Zest and juice of ½ lemon

Salt

¼ fennel bulb, thinly sliced, preferably on a mandoline

Small handful of fresh dill leaves, chopped

2 tablespoons sesame seeds, toasted (see page 100; optional)

2 tablespoons low-fat plain skyr or Cheater's Skyr (page 231)

Preheat the oven to 350°F. Line a baking sheet with parchment paper.

Place the salmon on the prepared baking sheet, skin-side down, and sprinkle with the cumin. Bake for about 12 minutes, or until just cooked through.

Meanwhile, bring a small saucepan of water to a boil. Add the peas and cook for 4 to 5 minutes, or until tender. Drain and let cool.

Put the avocado in a bowl and gently toss with the lemon zest and juice. Season lightly with salt. Add the fennel, peas, and dill. Transfer to a dinner plate and add the salmon. Sprinkle with the sesame seeds, if desired, and serve with the skyr on the side.

NOTE: If you are aiming for fewer calories, only use ½ avocado.

RATIO (Carb:Protein) = 1:4

PER SERVING: Calories 540 · Protein 27 g · Carbohydrate 7 g · Fiber 8 g · Fat 44 g · Saturated Fat 10 g · Sodium 130 mg

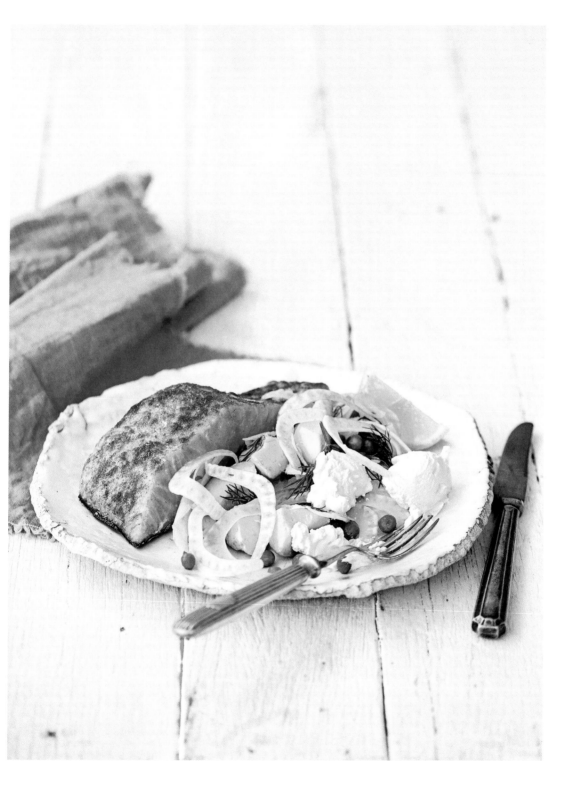

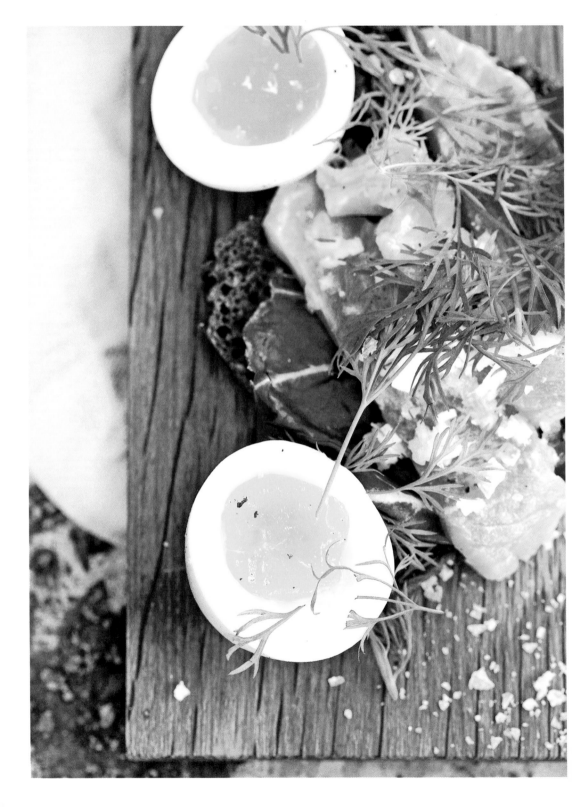

Open-Faced Sandwich with Salmon, Ginger & Lime

SERVES 1

If you can't be certain of the freshness of your salmon, substitute an equal amount of cured salmon, like gravlax or a mild Norwegian smoked salmon. It will be just as delicious.

4 ounces sushi-grade salmon fillet, thinly sliced across the grain

Salt and freshly ground black pepper

1 teaspoon finely chopped fresh ginger

Zest and juice of 1 lime

1 slice whole-grain rye bread or whole rye pumpernickel bread, toasted

3 bitter lettuce leaves, such as radicchio

1 large egg, hard-boiled and cut in half

Fresh dill sprigs, for serving

Place the salmon on a plate. Season with salt and pepper. Sprinkle with the ginger, lime zest, and lime juice.

Build your sandwich with the rye bread on the bottom, then the salmon, lettuce, egg, and dill on top.

RATIO (Carb:Protein) = 1:2

PER SERVING: Calories 414 · Protein 35 g · Carbohydrate 19 g · Fiber 4 g · Fat 21 g · Saturated Fat 6 g · Sodium 459 mg

Pork with Sage & Halloumi Filling

SERVES 1

Lean pork tenderloin cooks quickly, making it a good choice for weeknights. Sage and pear make this a perfect fall dish.

1 small fennel bulb, cut into wedges	Salt and freshly ground black pepper
½ red onion, cut into wedges	5 ounces pork tenderloin
1 small firm ripe pear, cored and cut into wedges	½ ounce (about 2 tablespoons) halloumi cheese
2 teaspoons balsamic vinegar	3 fresh sage leaves
Olive oil spray	1 cup packed arugula leaves

Preheat the oven to 350°F. Line a baking sheet with parchment paper.

Place the fennel, onion, and pear on the prepared baking sheet. Drizzle with 1 teaspoon of the balsamic vinegar, spray with olive oil spray, and season with salt and pepper. Bake for 10 minutes.

Meanwhile, use a sharp knife to cut a deep pocket in the side of the pork tenderloin, being careful not to cut all the way through. Place the halloumi cheese and sage in the pocket.

Coat a small nonstick skillet with olive oil spray and heat over high heat. Add the pork and cook for 1 to 2 minutes on each side or until golden. After the vegetables have cooked for 10 minutes, transfer the pork to the baking sheet and bake with the vegetables for 12 to 15 minutes, or until the pork is just cooked through and the vegetables are tender and golden. Transfer the pork to a plate, cover loosely with aluminum foil, and set aside for 3 minutes to rest.

Thickly slice the pork. Transfer to a plate. Add the vegetables and arugula, drizzle with the remaining balsamic vinegar, and serve.

RATIO (Carb:Protein) = 3:4

PER SERVING: Calories 376 • Protein 40 g • Carbohydrate 30 g • Fiber 10 g • Fat 10 g • Saturated Fat 3 g • Sodium 607 mg

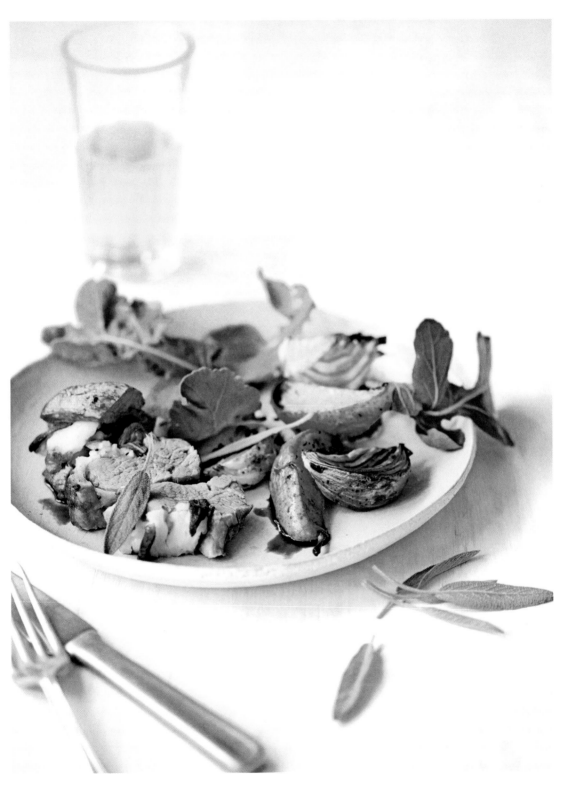

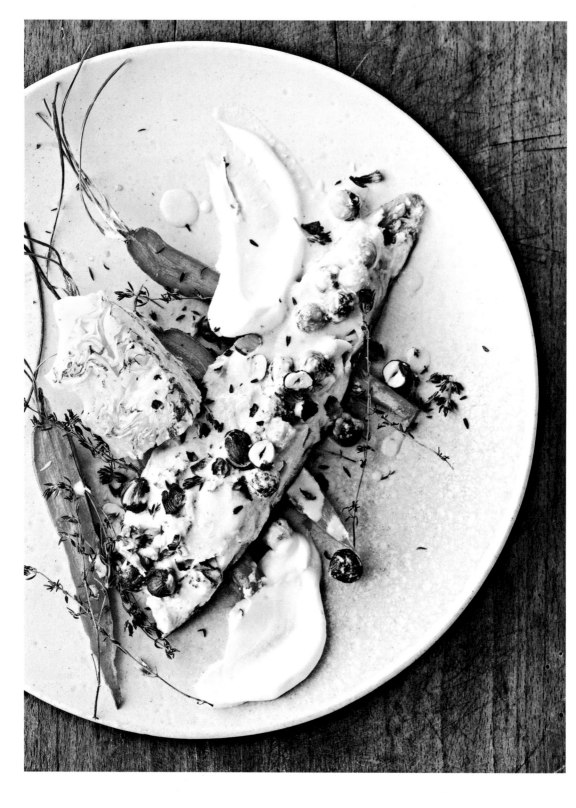

Cod with Carrot & Hazelnuts

SERVES 1

For fans of battered fried fish this all-in-one traybake meal offers a wholesome alternative, with chia seeds and hazelnuts providing the crunch, not doughy breading.

5 ounces skinless cod fillet

1 large egg white

1 tablespoon chia seeds or sesame seeds

Juice of ½ lemon

2 carrots, halved lengthwise

1 wedge green cabbage (about ⅛ small head)

Salt and freshly ground black pepper

5 sprigs fresh thyme

2 tablespoons low-fat plain skyr or Cheater's Skyr (page 231)

1 tablespoon coarsely chopped toasted hazelnuts (see page 80)

Preheat the oven to 400°F. Line a baking sheet with parchment paper.

Dip the cod in the egg white, roll in the chia seeds, and place on the prepared baking sheet. Drizzle with the lemon juice. Add the carrot halves and cabbage to the baking sheet. Season with salt and pepper. Scatter the thyme sprigs on top. Bake for 7 to 10 minutes, until the fish is cooked through.

Transfer the fish and vegetables to a plate, spread with the skyr, and top with the hazelnuts.

RATIO (Carb:Protein) = 2:3

PER SERVING: Calories 572 · Protein 35 g · Carbohydrate 23 g · Fiber 21 g · Fat 33 g · Saturated Fat 3 g · Sodium 460 mg

Citrus Chicken with
Roasted Sweet Potato & Arugula

SERVES 1

Low-GI sweet potatoes are a perfect foil for tangy-sweet chicken in a citrusy sauce.

1 small sweet potato (about 7 ounces), peeled and cut into 3/8-inch rounds

Olive oil spray

1/2 small red onion, thinly sliced

5 ounces boneless, skinless chicken breast, cut into 3/4-inch pieces

1 garlic clove, thinly sliced

1/4 cup fresh orange juice

1/2 teaspoon finely grated lemon zest

1 tablespoon fresh lemon juice

1/2 teaspoon wildflower honey

1 1/2 cups packed arugula leaves, for serving

Salt and freshly ground black pepper

Preheat the oven to 350°F. Line a baking sheet with parchment paper.

Place the sweet potato in a single layer on the prepared baking sheet and spray lightly with olive oil spray. Bake for 25 to 30 minutes, or until golden and tender.

Meanwhile, coat a large nonstick skillet with olive oil spray and heat over high heat. Add the onion and chicken and cook, stirring occasionally and turning the chicken, for 4 minutes, or until the chicken is golden brown. Add the garlic and cook for 30 seconds. Add the orange juice, lemon zest, lemon juice, and honey and simmer for 3 minutes, or until the chicken is cooked through and the sauce has reduced and become syrupy. Season with salt and pepper.

Serve the citrus chicken with the sweet potato and arugula.

RATIO (Carb:Protein) = 1:1

PER SERVING: Calories 448 · Protein 41 g · Carbohydrate 49 g · Fiber 8 g · Fat 8 g · Saturated Fat 2 g · Sodium 110 mg

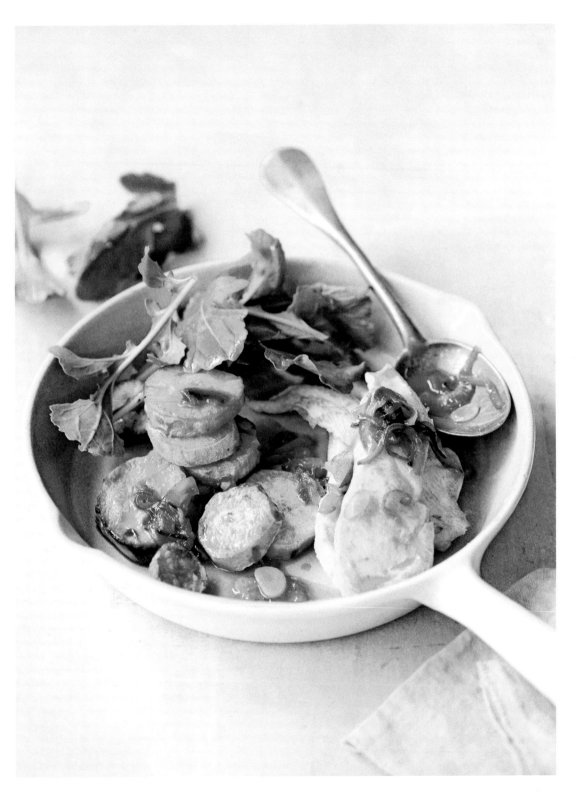

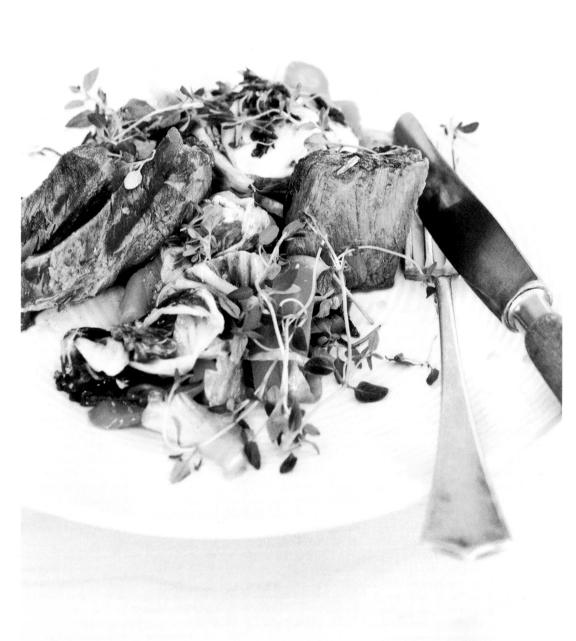

Veal Breast in Beer & Thyme

SERVES 2

Braising veal in beer gives it a tender texture and deep, rich flavor. This stew is a wonderful weekend dish that can be scaled up to serve a crowd.

2 teaspoons olive oil

1½ pounds veal breast on the bone

1 cup coarsely chopped seasonal vegetables, such as carrots

Handful of fresh thyme sprigs

1 teaspoon Dijon mustard

1 radicchio head, leaves separated

1 (12-ounce) bottle dark beer

2 cups water

Salt and freshly ground black pepper

1 slice low-GI whole-grain bread

Heat the olive oil in a heavy-bottomed medium saucepan over medium heat. Add the veal and cook, turning, until browned, about 5 minutes. Add the vegetables, half the thyme sprigs, and the mustard and sauté until the radicchio begins to wilt, about 2 minutes. Add the beer and water and bring to a simmer. Cover and simmer, stirring occasionally, for 1½ hours. Season with salt and pepper. Add the radicchio and cook another 10 minutes or until tender.

Use a slotted spoon to transfer to serving plates. Scatter the remaining thyme sprigs on top and serve with the bread alongside.

RATIO (Carb:Protein) = 1:2

PER SERVING: Calories 366 · Protein 38 g · Carbohydrate 35 g · Fiber 3 g · Fat 5 g · Saturated Fat 11 g · Sodium 707 mg

Chicken, Lentil & Swiss Chard Soup

SERVES 4

Make a batch—even a double batch—to eat for lunch or a simple supper throughout the coming week. It can also be frozen. This is quite high in protein so feel free to add a slice of low-GI bread.

2 teaspoons olive oil

1 large onion, chopped

2 carrots, diced

2 celery stalks, trimmed and diced

2 garlic cloves, crushed

1 teaspoon ground cumin

4 cups reduced-sodium chicken stock

2 cups water

2 boneless, skinless chicken breast halves, about 7 ounces each

1 cup green lentils

3 cups packed shredded Swiss chard leaves

Fresh lemon juice

Heat the olive oil in a large saucepan over medium heat. Add the onion, carrot, and celery and cook, stirring occasionally, for 5 to 6 minutes, or until softened. Add the garlic and cumin and cook for 1 minute more.

Add the stock and water and bring to a boil. Add the chicken. Reduce the heat to very low, cover, and simmer gently for 7 to 8 minutes, or until the chicken is just cooked through. Remove the chicken from the broth and let cool. Meanwhile, add the lentils to the pan and return to a boil, then reduce the heat to maintain a simmer and cook, partially covered, for 30 to 35 minutes, or until the lentils are tender, adding a little more water if it becomes too thick. Shred the cooled chicken and add it and the chard to the saucepan. Simmer for 5 minutes more. Add lemon juice to taste, and season with pepper.

Freeze any leftover soup in an airtight container or store in the refrigerator for 2 to 3 days.

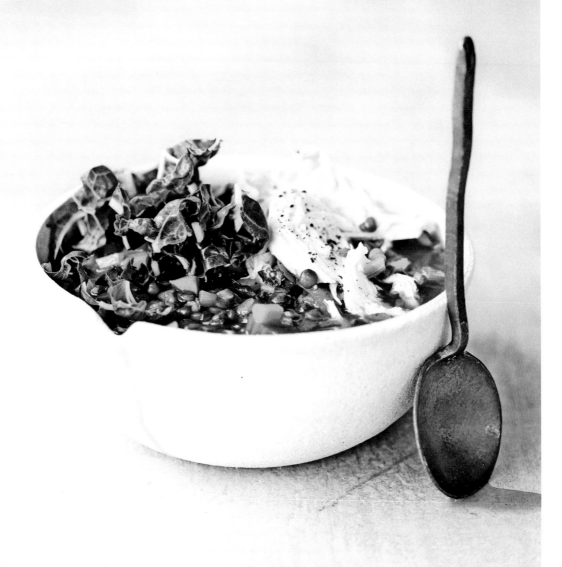

RATIO (Carb:Protein) = 1:3

PER SERVING: Calories 221 • Protein 29 g • Carbohydrate 12 g • Fiber 5 g • Fat 6 g •
Saturated Fat 1 g • Sodium 1,179 mg

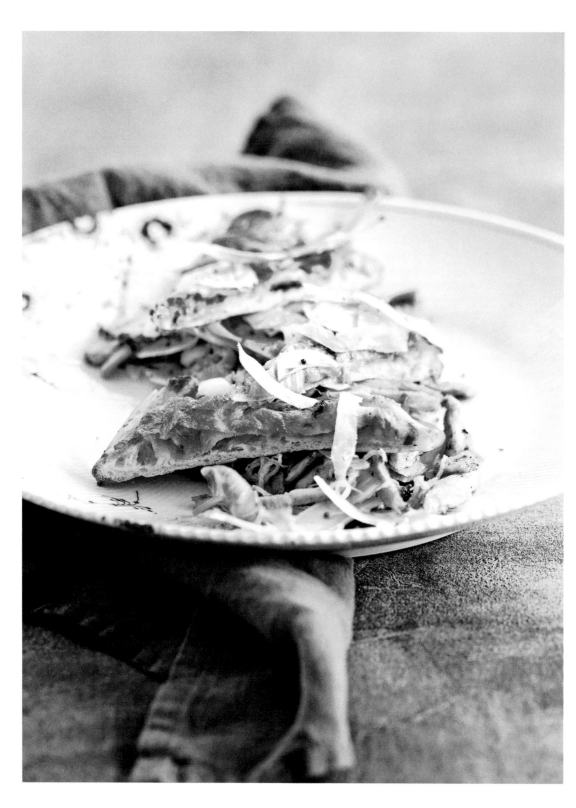

Pizza with Chicken & Greens

We said no food is excluded from our meal plan, and that includes pizza. Just look for a thin-crust, whole-grain variety with as few toppings as possible, and pile on the healthy veggies.

1 tablespoon olive oil

4 ounces boneless, skinless chicken breast

1 cup thinly sliced carrots, broccoli, or other seasonal vegetables

¼ fresh or frozen tomato-topped pizza (preferably whole wheat, with few other toppings)

Zest and juice of ½ lemon

Fresh basil leaves, for serving

Shaved Parmesan cheese, for serving

Preheat the oven to 400°F. Line a baking sheet or pizza pan with parchment paper.

Heat half the olive oil in a nonstick skillet over medium heat. Add the chicken and cook for 8 to 10 minutes, until cooked through. Transfer to a cutting board and cut into bite-size pieces.

Heat the remaining oil in the same pan. Add the vegetables and cook over medium heat until softened.

Put the pizza on the prepared baking sheet and bake as instructed on the package. Remove from the oven and sprinkle with the lemon zest and juice. Scatter the basil and cheese on top and serve with the chicken and vegetables.

RATIO (Carb:Protein) = 1:1 (estimated due to ingredient variations)

PER SERVING: Calories 718 · Protein 51 g · Carbohydrate 45 g · Fiber 14 g · Fat 35 g · Saturated Fat 10 g · Sodium 670 mg

Tuna with Wasabi, Cabbage, Almonds & Cucumber

SERVES 1

You'll get plenty of flavors, textures, and crunch in every bite of this pantry meal.

10 slices seedless (English) cucumber

½ teaspoon wasabi paste, or more if desired

¼ green cabbage, thinly sliced

Thinly sliced zest and juice ½ lemon

1 (2.6-ounce) package tuna in water, drained

2 tablespoons coarsely chopped toasted almonds (see page 99)

Low-fat plain skyr or Cheater's Skyr (page 231), for serving (optional)

Mix the cucumber, soy sauce, and wasabi in a small bowl.

Place the cabbage in a wide soup bowl and sprinkle with the lemon zest and juice. Add the cucumber mixture, tuna, almonds, and a dollop of skyr, if desired.

RATIO (Carb:Protein) = 1:2 (without skyr)

PER SERVING: Calories 367 · Protein 34 g · Carbohydrate 17 g · Fiber 10 g · Fat 16 g · Saturated Fat 2 g · Sodium 1,754 mg

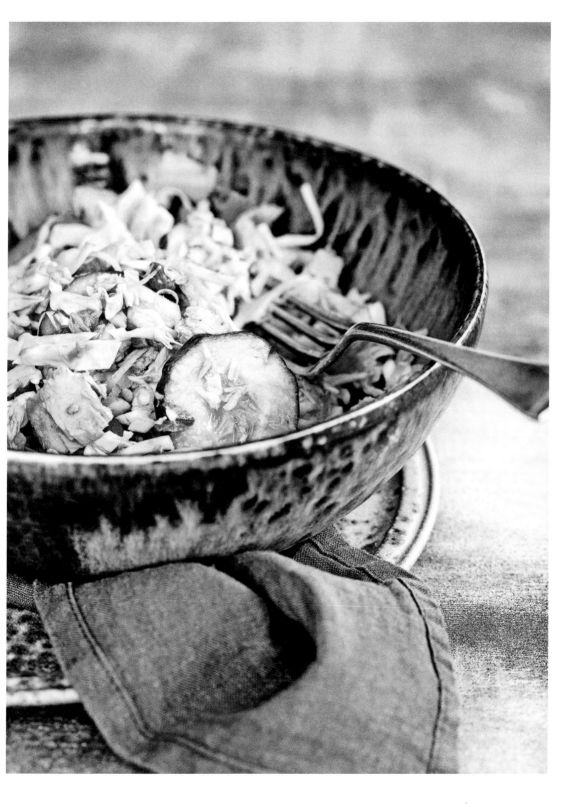

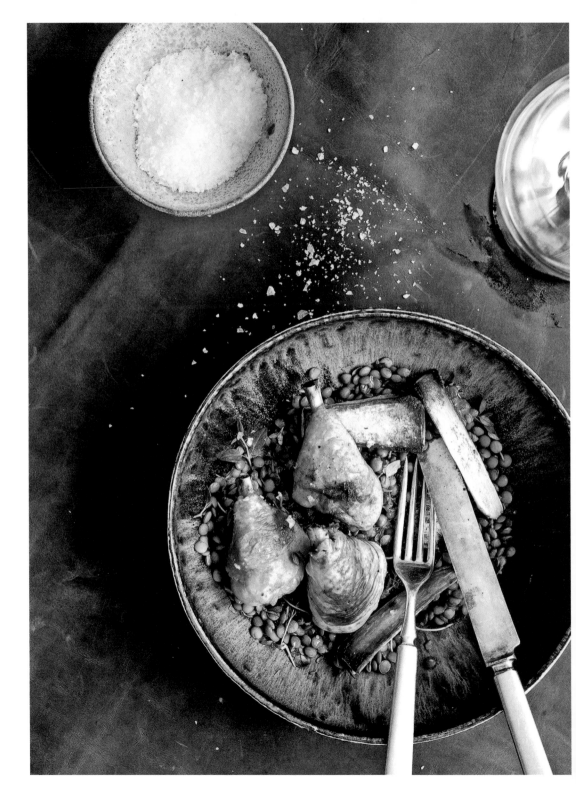

Chicken Drumsticks with Fennel & Lentils

SERVES 1

Danish chickens tend to be smaller than those in the United States; two medium drumsticks would be an equivalent portion. This is a meal you could easily serve to guests or family with no explanations or excuses required.

2 medium or 3 very small chicken drumsticks

1 teaspoon ground fennel seeds

Salt

1 parsnip, peeled and quartered lengthwise

Olive oil spray

½ cup green lentils

1 tablespoon honey

1 tablespoon Dijon mustard

Juice of 1 lime

1 teaspoon fresh thyme leaves

Preheat the oven to 350°F. Line a baking sheet with parchment paper.

Rub the fennel over the chicken and sprinkle with salt. Place on the prepared baking sheet with the parsnips and spray with olive oil spray. Bake for 40 minutes, or until the chicken is cooked through and the parsnip is tender.

Meanwhile, bring a medium saucepan of water to a boil over medium-high heat. Add the lentils and cook for 12 to 14 minutes, or until just tender. Drain and rinse under cold water to cool. Put the lentils in a bowl and mix in the honey, mustard, lime juice, and thyme.

Serve the chicken and parsnip with the lentils alongside.

RATIO (Carb:Protein) = 1:1

PER SERVING: Calories 307 · Protein 55 g · Carbohydrate 48 g · Fiber 11 g · Fat 30 g · Saturated Fat 8 g · Sodium 674 mg

Salmon Meatballs with Chickpeas & Cabbage

SERVES 1

If you have an aebelskiver pan, used to make a traditional doughnut hole–like Scandinavian treat, use it to cook the meatballs; the round indentations will make turning the delicate fish balls a breeze.

¾ cup canned chickpeas, drained and rinsed

5 ounces skinless salmon fillet, finely chopped

Zest and juice of 1 lime

1 large egg, beaten

1 tablespoon finely chopped fresh ginger

1 teaspoon minced seeded fresh red chile, such as Fresno or jalapeño

Salt and freshly ground black pepper

2 teaspoons olive oil

¼ green cabbage, chopped

2 fresh dill sprigs

½ cup low-fat plain skyr or Cheater's Skyr (page 231)

1 teaspoon ground cumin

Finely chop the chickpeas. Transfer to a bowl and add the salmon, lime zest, all but 1 teaspoon of the lime juice, egg, ginger, and chile. Season with salt and black pepper and mix well. Roll the mixture into 6 meatballs.

Heat the olive oil in a skillet over medium heat. Add the meatballs and fry, turning occasionally, for 6 to 8 minutes, or until cooked through. Transfer to a plate and cover to keep warm.

Add the cabbage to the skillet. Add the reserved lime juice and the dill, and season with salt and black pepper. Cook over medium heat for about 5 minutes, or until the cabbage softens.

Mix the skyr and cumin in a small bowl and season with salt.

Serve the salmon meatballs with the cabbage and a dollop of the cumin cream.

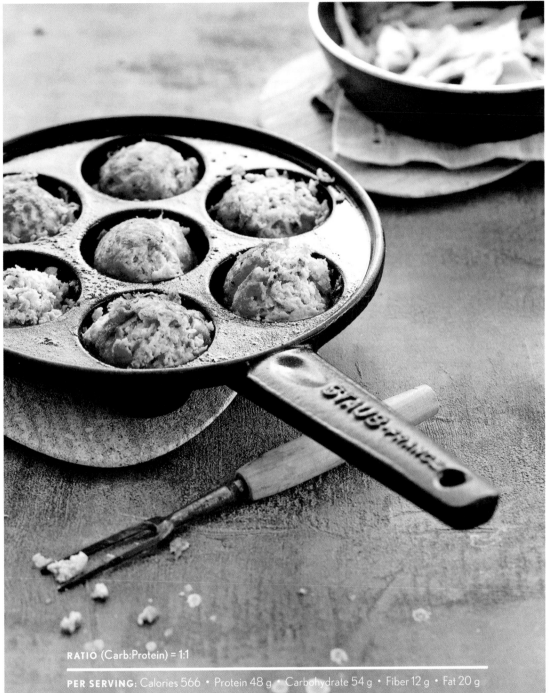

RATIO (Carb:Protein) = 1:1
_____

PER SERVING: Calories 566 • Protein 48 g • Carbohydrate 54 g • Fiber 12 g • Fat 20 g • Saturated Fat 8 g • Sodium 764 mg

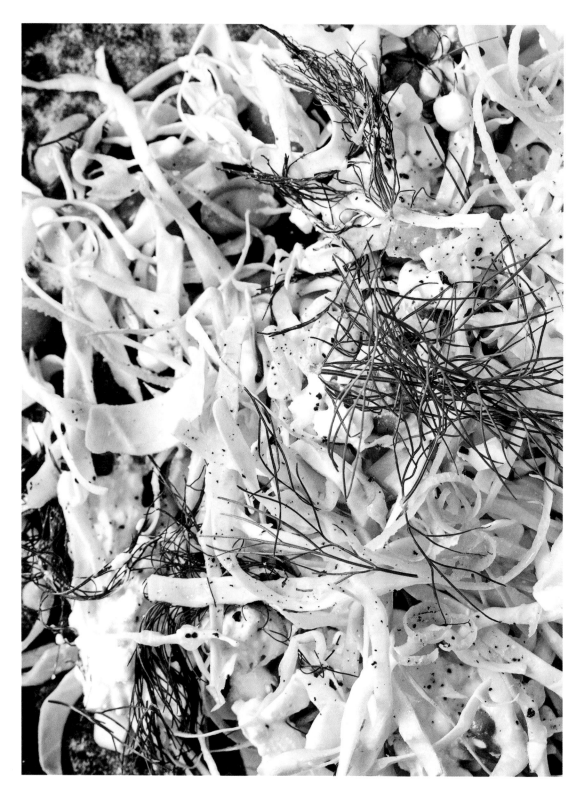

Edamame with Cabbage & Dill

SERVES 1

Meatless entrées don't have to be low in protein, as this mix of greens and dairy sweetened with a touch of honey demonstrates. Dill and lemon zest keep it from being bland.

½ cup cottage cheese

1 tablespoon pure wildflower honey

1 teaspoon finely chopped fresh dill, or more to taste

Zest and juice of ½ lemon

Salt and freshly ground black pepper

¼ green cabbage, cored and shredded

⅔ cup thawed frozen shelled edamame

Mix together the cottage cheese, honey, dill, lemon zest, and lemon juice in a small bowl. Season with salt and pepper.

Combine the cabbage and edamame in a serving bowl, fold in the cottage cheese, and serve.

RATIO (Carb:Protein) = 1:1

PER SERVING: Calories 274 · Protein 21 g · Carbohydrate 46 g · Fiber 11 g · Fat 3 g · Saturated Fat 4 g · Sodium 481 mg

Pasta Bolognese

SERVES 2

A hearty dish made even more rib-sticking with lentils and earthy celery root. Just 1½ ounces of pasta per serving provides all the satisfaction with a fraction of the carbs.

Olive oil spray

9 ounces lean ground beef

1 onion, chopped

1 carrot, chopped

1 garlic clove, finely chopped

2 (14-ounce) cans diced tomatoes

Salt and freshly ground black pepper

½ cup green lentils

3 ounces whole wheat pasta

1 tomato, cut into wedges

1 tablespoon olive oil

Juice of ½ lemon

2 tablespoons freshly grated Parmesan cheese

½ cup grated peeled celery root (celeriac)

Coat a skillet with olive oil spray and heat over medium-high heat. Add the beef, onion, carrot, and garlic and cook, stirring often, for 6 to 8 minutes, or until the meat is browned. Add the tomatoes with their juices and bring to a boil. Reduce the heat to low and simmer, uncovered, for 20 minutes, or until the sauce thickens. Season with salt and pepper.

Meanwhile, bring a medium saucepan of water to a boil over medium-high heat. Add the lentils and cook for 12 to 14 minutes, or until the lentils are just tender. Drain and rinse under cold water to cool.

Bring a second saucepan of salted water to a boil over high heat. Add the pasta and cook according to the package directions until al dente. Drain well.

Mix the lentils, tomato, oil, lemon juice, and a pinch of salt together in a small bowl.

Serve the meat sauce over the pasta, sprinkled with cheese and celery root, with the lentil salad alongside. Or, as a variation, mix the lentil mixture into the meat sauce and sprinkle with the celery root; serve with the cheese on the side.

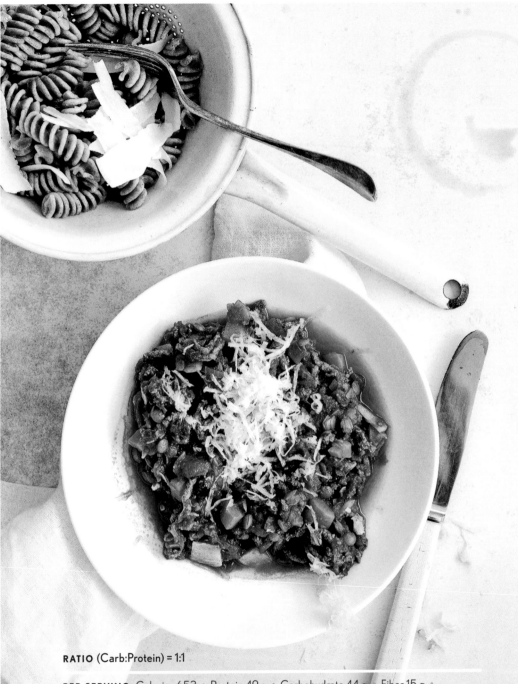

RATIO (Carb:Protein) = 1:1

PER SERVING: Calories 653 · Protein 49 g · Carbohydrate 44 g · Fiber 15 g · Fat 28 g · Saturated Fat 9 g · Sodium 539 mg

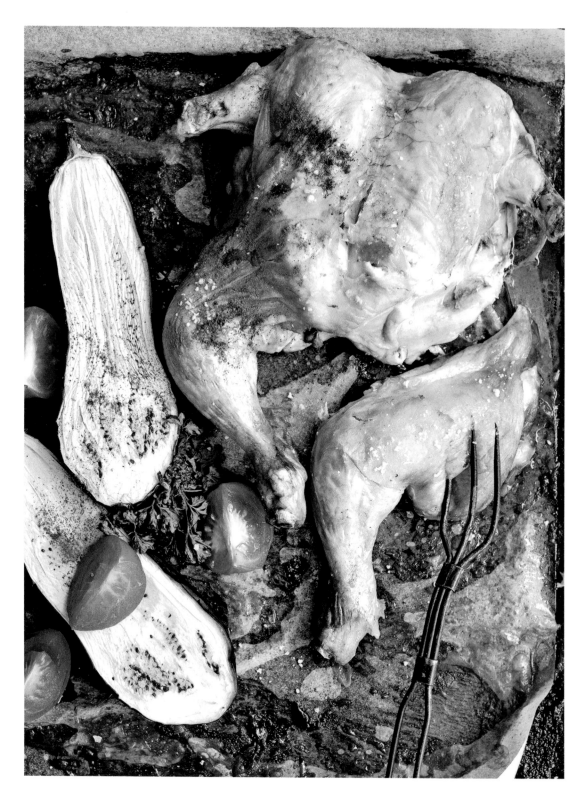

Chicken with Eggplant, Tomato & Cinnamon

SERVES 4

Cinnamon is a powerful antioxidant, and it lends its warming qualities to a simple roast chicken served on a bed of creamy roasted eggplant.

Olive oil spray

1 whole chicken (about 3 pounds)

Salt

1 teaspoon ground cinnamon

1 narrow eggplant, halved lengthwise

Small handful of fresh parsley leaves, chopped

½ cup low-fat plain skyr or Cheater's Skyr (page 231)

1 tablespoon olive oil

Preheat the oven to 400°F. Coat a roasting pan with olive oil spray.

Use a long sharp knife or poultry scissors to cut out the backbone of the chicken and discard. With the skin side facing up, press down hard on the chicken breast to flatten. Season with salt and the cinnamon. Place in the prepared roasting pan and bake for 50 to 55 minutes, or until the chicken shows no sign of pink when pierced at the drumstick joint.

Meanwhile, sprinkle the eggplant with salt and let drain in a colander for 20 minutes to remove the bitter juices. Rinse and pat dry. Add the eggplant halves to the pan with the chicken for the last 20 to 30 minutes to roast until tender.

Discard the eggplant skin and process the flesh in a blender until smooth. Transfer to a small bowl and fold in the parsley and skyr. Drizzle with the olive oil.

Serve the chicken with the eggplant puree and tomato wedges alongside.

RATIO (Carb:Protein) = 1:12

PER SERVING: Calories 607 · Protein 61 g · Carbohydrate 5 g · Fiber 3 g · Fat 38 g · Saturated Fat 11 g · Sodium 240 mg

Chia-Crusted Tofu with Tomato, Spinach & Green Bean Rice

SERVES 1

Those who object to the texture of tofu may be swayed by this colorful meat-less stir-fry. A coating of chia seeds adds crunch and color to the tofu.

2 teaspoons black chia seeds

4 ounces firm tofu, cut lengthwise into four slices

Olive oil spray

6 cherry tomatoes, halved

⅓ cup thinly sliced green beans

¾ cup cooked low-GI basmati rice

1 cup packed baby spinach leaves

2 teaspoons reduced-sodium soy sauce

1 teaspoon toasted sesame oil

Place the chia seeds on a small plate. Press one long side of each piece of tofu in the seeds to coat. Set aside.

Coat a large nonstick skillet with olive oil spray and heat over high heat. Add the tomatoes and green beans and cook, stirring occasionally, for 2 to 3 minutes, or until the beans are crisp-tender. Add the rice and spinach and cook for 1 to 2 minutes, or until the rice is heated through and the spinach just wilts. Stir in the soy sauce, then transfer to a bowl and cover to keep warm.

Wipe the pan clean, spray with a little more olive oil spray, and return to high heat. Cook the tofu for 2 minutes on each side, or until the uncoated side is golden. Serve the tofu with the rice mixture alongside.

RATIO (Carb:Protein) = 2:1

PER SERVING: Calories 468 · Protein 24 g · Carbohydrate 42 g · Fiber 16 g · Fat 19 g · Saturated Fat 3 g · Sodium 429 mg

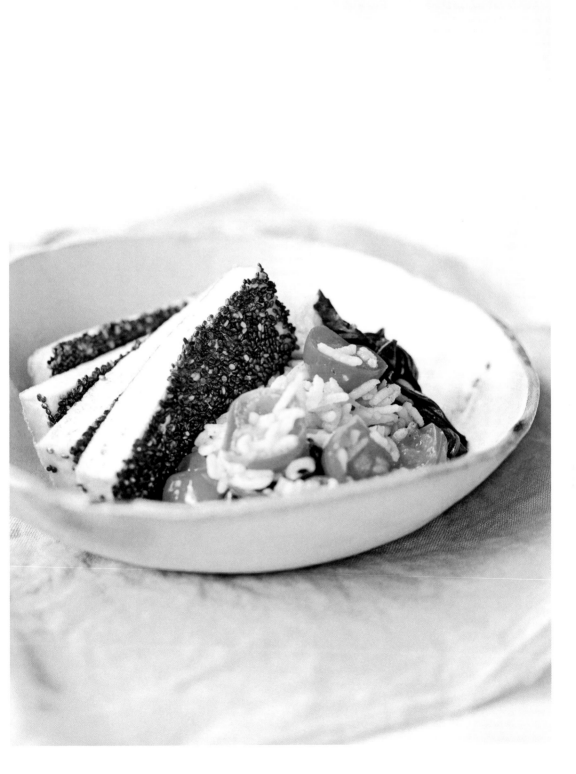

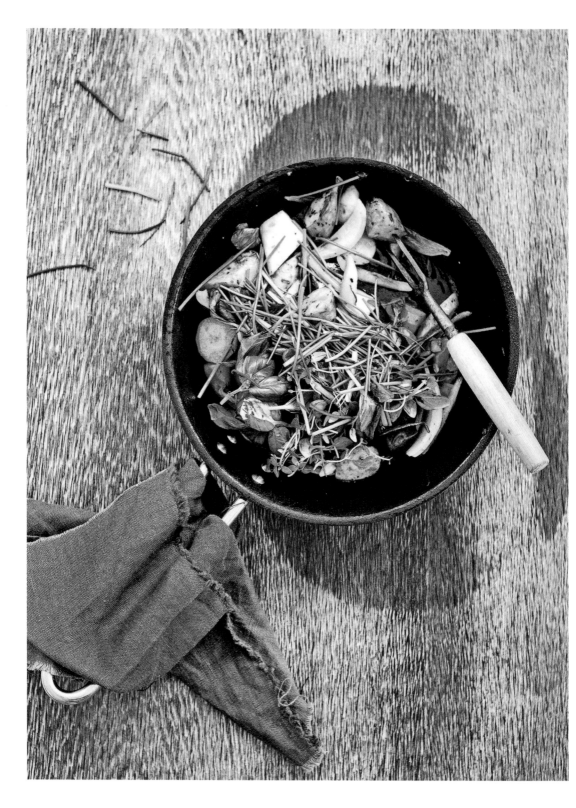

Sauté of Root Vegetables with Chorizo

SERVES 1

Precooked sausages are the weeknight cook's ace in the hole. Tossed with pan-roasted vegetables and a generous amount of herbs, they offer long-cooked flavor in less than 15 minutes.

3½ ounces smoked chorizo or precooked pork, chicken, or turkey sausage

Olive oil spray

1 small carrot, cut into ½-inch rounds

1 small parsnip, peeled and cut into ½-inch rounds

¼ onion, cut into thin wedges

Coarse salt

Handful of mixed fresh herb leaves, such as parsley, chives, and thyme

Coat a nonstick skillet with olive oil spray and heat over medium-high heat. Add the chorizo and cook, turning occasionally, for 2 minutes, or until beginning to brown. Add the vegetables, reduce the heat to medium-low, and cook, stirring often, for 8 to 10 minutes, or until the chorizo is heated through and the vegetables are softened slightly. Thickly slice the chorizo and return it to the pan. Toss to combine with the vegetables.

Season with salt, sprinkle with the herbs, and serve.

RATIO (Carb:Protein) = 1:2

PER SERVING: Calories 331 · Protein 19 g · Carbohydrate 11 g · Fiber 6 g · Fat 23 g · Saturated Fat 7 g · Sodium 832 mg

Shrimp with Chile, Grapefruit & Cabbage

SERVES 1

Although clearly not a traditional Scandinavian dish, with its piquant accents of chile, soy, and fish sauce, this stir-fry is both vividly colored and flavored, nice for those days when your taste buds need a jolt.

2 teaspoons olive oil

1 cup thinly sliced red cabbage

½ red onion, thinly sliced

4 ounces peeled and deveined small shrimp

½ fresh red chile, such as Fresno or jalapeño, seeded and thinly sliced

½ pink grapefruit, peeled and cut into wedges

1 tablespoon toasted sliced almonds (see page 99)

1 tablespoon soy sauce

1 tablespoon fish sauce

Freshly ground black pepper

Heat the olive oil in a wok over high heat. Add the cabbage and onion and cook, stirring continuously, until softened, about 2 minutes. Add the shrimp and chile. Cook for 2 to 3 minutes, until the shrimp turn opaque. Add the grapefruit, almonds, soy sauce, fish sauce, and pepper and toss to combine.

RATIO (Carb:Protein) = 1:2

PER SERVING: Calories 333 · Protein 29 g · Carbohydrate 12 g · Fiber 7 g · Fat 17 g · Saturated Fat 2 g · Sodium 2,905 mg

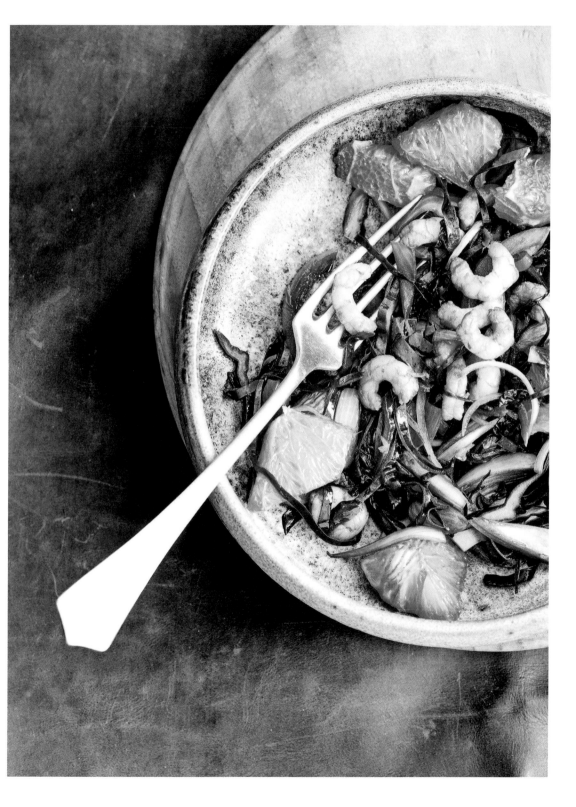

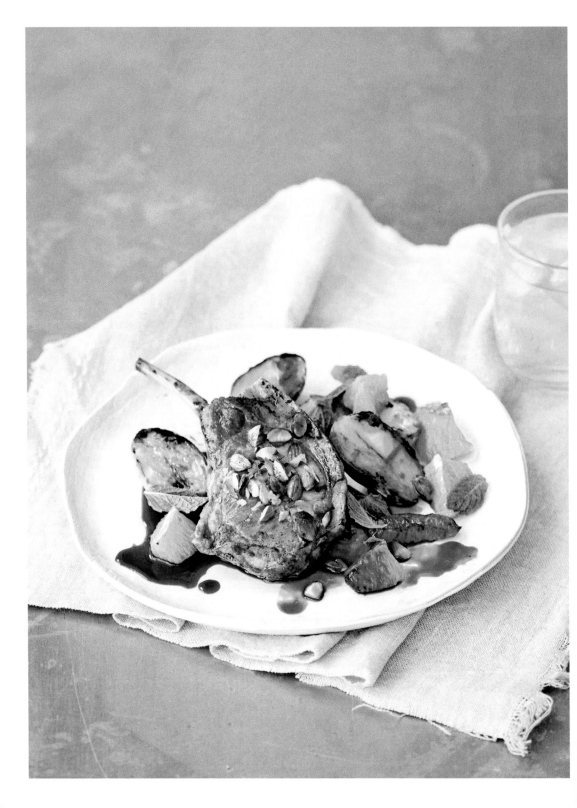

Pork Chop with Mint, Potato & Orange

SERVES 1

Pork pairs especially well with tart/sweet/salty sauces like this one. For an elegant presentation ask your butcher to "French" the bone.

Olive oil spray

1 bone-in, center-cut loin pork chop (about 7 ounces)

½ blood orange, peeled and cut into wedges

10 large fresh mint sprigs, plus leaves for serving

2 small fingerling potatoes, boiled and cut into wedges

Salt and freshly ground black pepper

2 teaspoons wildflower honey

2 teaspoons soy sauce

1 tablespoon chopped almonds

Preheat the oven to 350°F. Line a baking sheet with parchment paper.

Coat a nonstick skillet with olive oil spray and heat over medium-high heat. Add the pork and cook, turning once, for about 4 minutes, or until browned on both sides.

Place the orange wedges, mint sprigs, and potato on the prepared baking sheet and season with salt and pepper. Place the pork on top. Drizzle with the honey and soy sauce and sprinkle with the almonds. Bake until the pork reaches 145°F on an instant-read thermometer, about 12 minutes. Sprinkle with the mint leaves and serve.

RATIO (Carb:Protein) = 1:1

PER SERVING: Calories 407 · Protein 53 g · Carbohydrate 43 g · Fiber 8 g · Fat 9 g · Saturated Fat 1 g · Sodium 930 mg

Chicken, Cabbage & Curry Wrap

SERVES 1

The Nordic Way is all about ratios, and this wrap stands the usual wrap-to-filling ratio on its head, with a plenty of fresh vegetables and a curry sauce to bolster the chicken.

1 boneless, skinless chicken breast half (about 6 ounces)

1 whole wheat flour tortilla

1 cup finely shredded green cabbage

½ carrot, very thinly sliced

½ green bell pepper, seeded and thinly sliced

2 small cauliflower florets, broken into very small pieces

Salt and freshly ground black pepper

Zest and juice of ½ lemon

1 tablespoon curry powder

1 teaspoon hot pepper sauce

½ cup low-fat plain skyr or Cheater's Skyr (page 231)

Preheat the oven to 400°F. Line a baking sheet with parchment paper.

Place the chicken on the prepared baking sheet and bake for 15 to 17 minutes, until it reaches 165°F on an instant-read thermometer. Transfer to a cutting board and let cool for 5 minutes. Cut crosswise into thin slices.

Meanwhile, warm the tortilla on the rack in the oven for a few minutes.

Combine the cabbage, carrot, bell pepper, cauliflower, lemon zest, and lemon juice in a medium bowl. Season with salt and pepper.

Toast the curry powder in a small nonstick skillet over medium heat, stirring often, for about 1 minute, or until aromatic. Sprinkle the curry powder and hot sauce over the sliced chicken.

Spread the tortilla with the skyr, add the cabbage mixture and sliced chicken, and roll into a wrap.

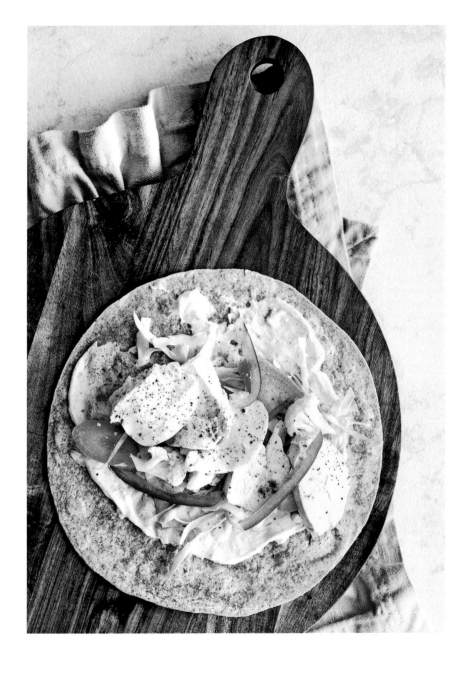

RATIO (Carb:Protein) = 1:2

PER SERVING: Calories 453 • Protein 67 g • Carbohydrate 28 g • Fiber 13 g • Fat 5 g •
Saturated Fat 1 g • Sodium 482 mg

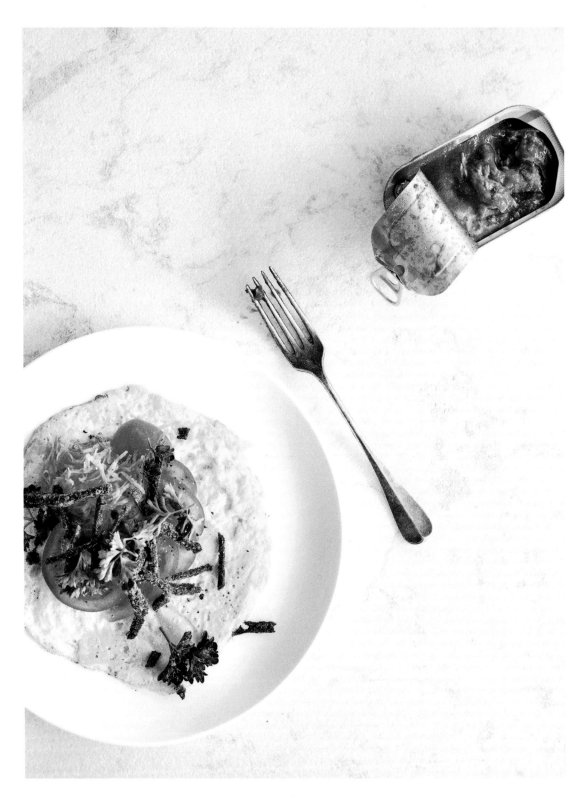

Omelet with Mackerel, Tomatoes & Rye Bread

SERVES 1

While this technically falls into the category of Breakfast for Dinner, it would indeed make a very sustaining (and sustainable) breakfast!

Olive oil spray

2 large eggs, lightly whisked

1 tomato, sliced

1 small carrot, grated

1 slice whole-grain rye bread or whole rye pumpernickel bread, toasted and cut into thin strips

Fresh parsley leaves

Salt and freshly ground black pepper

1 (2.25-ounce) can mackerel or sardines in tomato sauce

Coat a nonstick skillet with olive oil spray and heat over medium heat. Add the eggs and cook until the whites have set, then flip them over. Cook for 30 seconds more to set the yolks and transfer to a plate.

Top with the tomato, carrot, rye strips, and parsley. Season with salt and pepper and serve with the mackerel alongside.

RATIO (Carb:Protein) = 1:1

PER SERVING: Calories 476 · Protein 35 g · Carbohydrate 27 g · Fiber 8 g · Fat 24 g · Saturated Fat 6 g · Sodium 888 mg

Salmon with Herbs, Quick Cucumber Pickle & Egg

SERVES 1

Salmon, dill, eggs, and cucumber are fundamentals of the Scandinavian kitchen, and for good reason; not only do they provide superior nutrition, but their flavors can be combined in infinite ways. Here the cucumber is pickled, enlivening the mild poached salmon.

Salt

⅓ cup rye berries or pearl barley

4 ounces salmon fillet

Mixed dried or fresh herbs, such as chives, dill, and parsley leaves

¼ seedless (English) cucumber, coarsely chopped

½ cup apple cider vinegar

Leaves from 4 sprigs fresh parsley

1 large egg, hard-boiled and halved

Bring a medium saucepan of salted water to a boil over high heat. Add the rye and reduce the heat to medium. Cook the rye until it is tender, 20 to 30 minutes. Drain in a sieve, rinse under cold running water, and let cool.

Meanwhile, fill a skillet halfway with water and bring to the boil over medium heat. Add the salmon and place the herbs on top. Reduce the heat to low. Cover and simmer for 5 to 7 minutes, until the salmon is rosy pink when flaked in the center. Using a slotted spatula, transfer to paper towels to drain.

While the salmon is cooking, bring the vinegar to a boil in a small saucepan. Put the cucumber in a small bowl, sprinkle with salt, and pour in the hot vinegar. Set aside for 5 minutes, then drain. Mix with the drained rye and parsley in a medium bowl.

Place the salmon on a dinner plate, top with the cucumber mixture, and serve with the egg alongside.

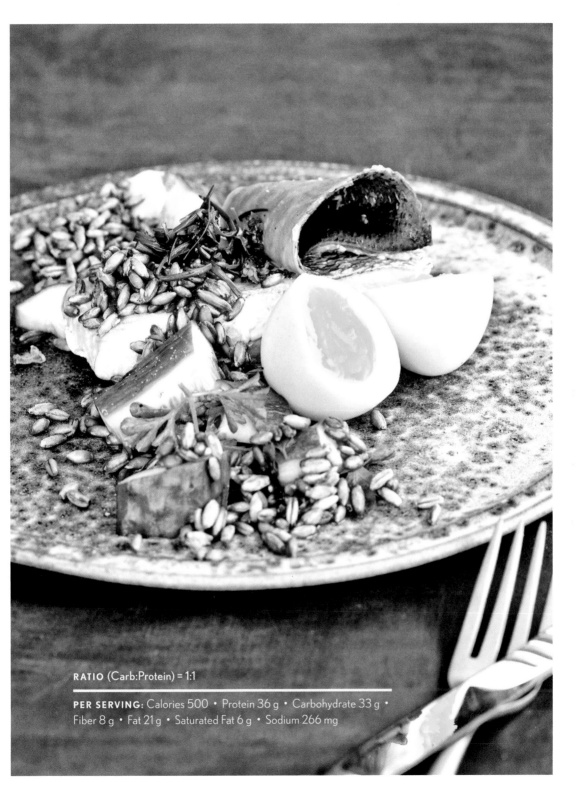

RATIO (Carb:Protein) = 1:1

PER SERVING: Calories 500 • Protein 36 g • Carbohydrate 33 g • Fiber 8 g • Fat 21 g • Saturated Fat 6 g • Sodium 266 mg

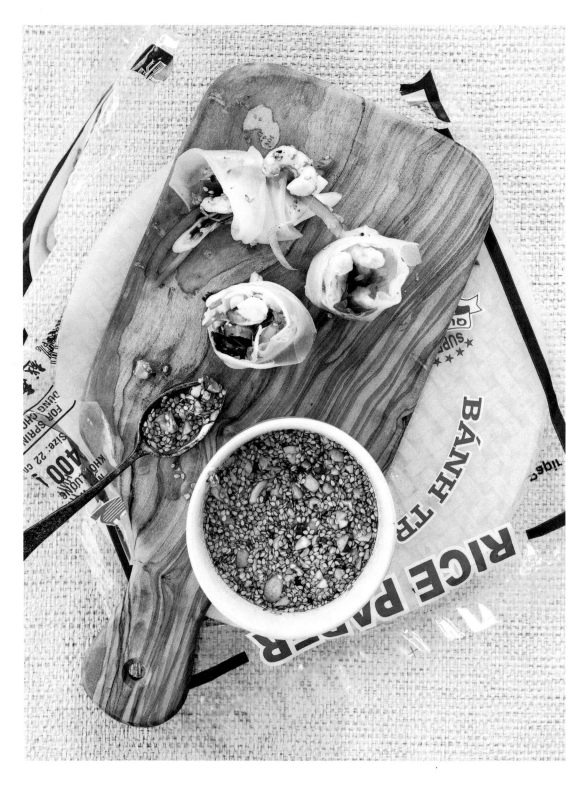

Rice Paper Rolls with Shrimp

SERVES 2

Foods familiar to the Nordic table—shrimp and fennel—get a Southeast Asian gloss in these attractive summer rolls. The sesame dressing adds a pop of sweet/hot/umami flavor.

3½ ounces small cooked shrimp

1 scallion, white and green parts thinly sliced

½ green bell pepper, seeded and cut into thin strips

2 fresh basil leaves, shredded

½ fennel bulb, cored and outer layer removed, very thinly sliced

4 (8-inch) rounds Thai or Vietnamese rice paper

SESAME DRESSING

1 tablespoon sesame seeds

1 tablespoon fish sauce

1 tablespoon wildflower honey

½ fresh red chile, seeded and finely chopped

1 teaspoon chopped salted peanuts

1 teaspoon peanut oil

Salt and freshly ground black pepper

Mix the shrimp, scallion, bell pepper, fennel, and basil in a bowl.

For each roll, soak a rice paper round in a bowl of warm water for a few seconds, just until it softens. Transfer to a folded kitchen towel to drain. Place one-quarter of the mixture on the round. Fold in each side about 1 inch, then roll up the round from the bottom.

To make the sesame dressing: Whisk the sesame seeds, fish sauce, honey, lime juice, chile, peanuts, and peanut oil together in a small bowl. Season with salt and pepper.

Serve the rolls with the sesame dressing for dipping.

RATIO (Carb:Protein) = 1:1

PER SERVING: Calories 237 · Protein 16 g · Carbohydrate 18 g · Fiber 4 g · Fat 11 g · Saturated Fat 2 g · Sodium 1,163 mg

Cod & Tomato Salad

Any mild white fish can stand in for cod here. If you don't love cooking fish, this streamlined baking technique may win you over.

Salt

⅓ cup rye berries or pearl barley

10 fresh mint leaves

5 ounces cod fillet

1 tomato, sliced

¼ small red onion, sliced

Fresh parsley, for serving

1 tablespoon assorted olives, for serving

Freshly ground black pepper

Preheat the oven to 400°F. Line a baking sheet with parchment paper.

Bring a medium saucepan of salted water to a boil over medium heat. Add the rye and cook for 20 to 30 minutes, or until the grains are tender. Drain and rinse. Transfer to a bowl and toss with the mint leaves. Season with salt.

Meanwhile, place the cod on the prepared baking sheet and bake for 10 minutes, or until cooked through.

Transfer the cod to a plate and add the rye mixture, tomato, onion, parsley, and olives. Season with salt and pepper and serve.

RATIO (Carb:Protein) = 1:1

PER SERVING: Calories 397 · Protein 36 g · Carbohydrate 41 g · Fiber 13 g · Fat 7 g · Saturated Fat <1 g · Sodium 630 mg

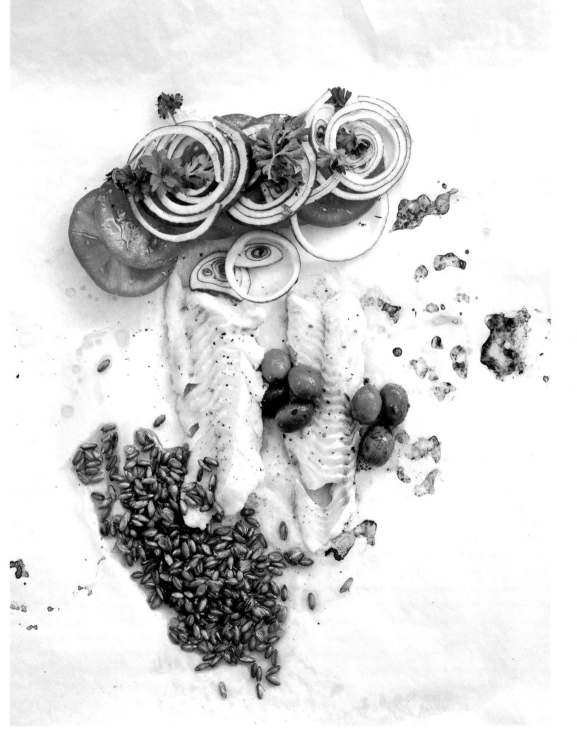

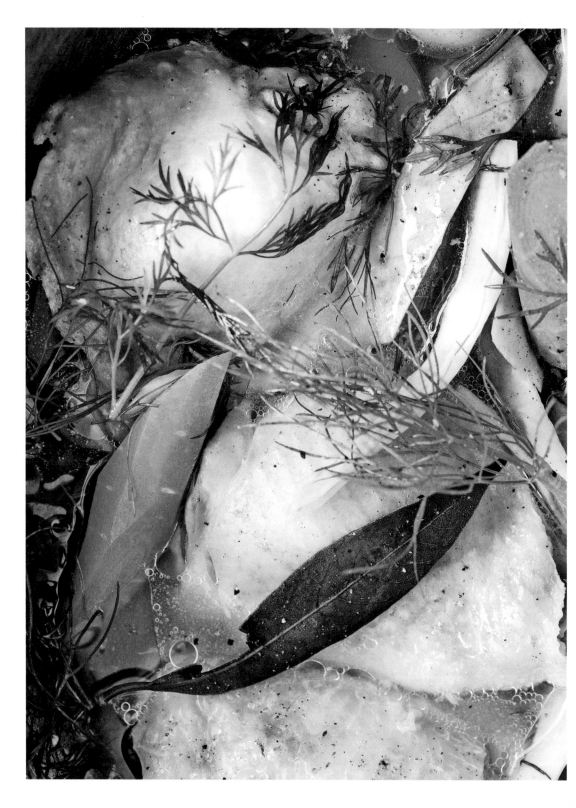

Chicken with Carrots & Potatoes

SERVES 1

Yet another way to combine staples of the Nordic pantry into a homespun but soothing dish. Here the chicken and vegetables are simmered in a lightly juice-sweetened poaching liquid rather than stewed.

2 chicken drumsticks or
  bone-in thighs

2 small carrots, thickly sliced

3 bay leaves

½ cup apple juice

4 small fingering potatoes,
  halved

¼ green cabbage, thinly sliced

3 fresh dill sprigs

Salt and freshly ground black
  pepper

Place the chicken, carrots, and bay leaves in a medium saucepan. Add the apple juice and enough cold water to cover. Bring to a simmer over medium heat. Reduce the heat to medium-low and simmer for 30 minutes.

Add the potatoes and simmer for 10 minutes more. Add the cabbage and dill and cook for 3 minutes more. Season with salt and pepper.

Drain the chicken and vegetables. Discard the bay leaves and, if desired, the chicken skin. Serve.

RATIO (Carb:Protein) = 2:1

PER SERVING: Calories 582 · Protein 44 g · Carbohydrate 82 g · Fiber 14 g · Fat 12 g · Saturated Fat 5 g · Sodium 370 mg

Spicy Beef & Noodle Lettuce Wraps

Yet another illustration of how readily the principles of The Nordic Way can be applied to foods in your favorite ethnic traditions. These beef bundles get a hint of Southeast Asia from rice noodles and lemongrass.

2 ounces bean thread noodles

Boiling water, as needed, for the noodles

Olive oil spray

4 ounces trimmed beef sirloin steak

1 fresh red chile, such as Fresno or jalapeño, seeded and finely chopped

1 teaspoon finely chopped lemongrass

1 garlic clove, crushed

3½ ounces snow peas, trimmed and halved crosswise

¼ red bell pepper, seeded and thinly sliced

2 teaspoons fresh lime juice

1 tablespoon chopped fresh cilantro, plus more for serving

Baby lettuce leaves, for serving

Place the noodles in a medium heatproof bowl, cover with boiling water, and set aside for 3 to 4 minutes, or just until softened. Drain well.

Meanwhile, coat a wok with olive oil spray and heat over high heat. Add the beef and sear for 2 minutes each side, or until cooked to medium-rare. Transfer to a plate and set aside. Add the chile, lemongrass, and garlic to the wok and stir-fry for 30 seconds. Add the snow peas and bell pepper and stir-fry for 2 minutes more, or until crisp-tender.

Return the beef to the wok and add the noodles, lime juice, and cilantro. Toss to combine. Spoon the mixture into the lettuce leaves, scatter with cilantro, and serve immediately.

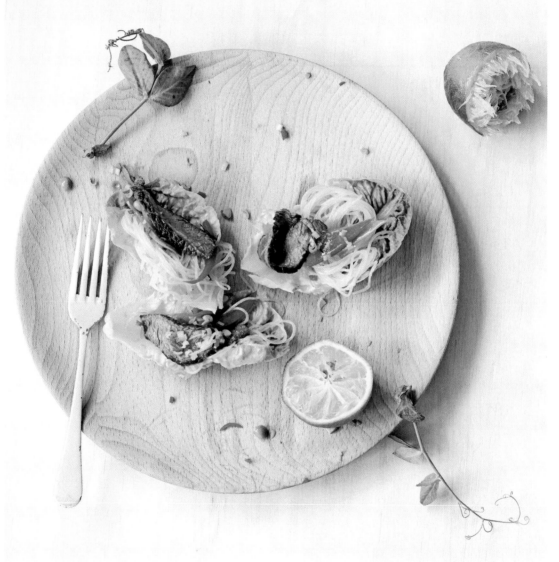

RATIO (Carb:Protein) = 1:1

PER SERVING: Calories 315 • Protein 29 g • Carbohydrate 21 g • Fiber 7 g • Fat 11 g • Saturated Fat 3 g • Sodium 69 mg

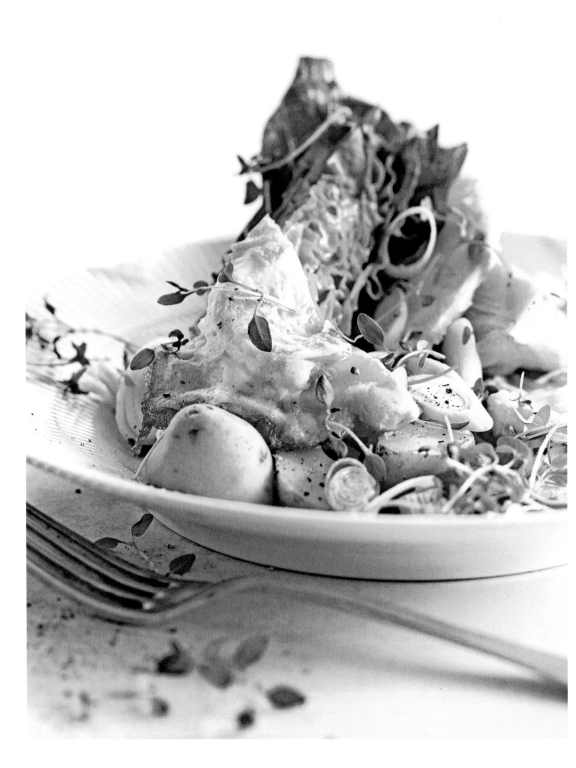

Potatoes with Eggs & Lettuce

SERVES 1

Here's a low-GI side for your next cookout. Pair it with a vinegar-based slaw.

½ head baby lettuce, leaves
separated

2 small fingerling potatoes,
boiled and halved

1 scallion, white and green parts
thinly sliced

Mixed fresh herbs, such as
thyme and parsley

1 tablespoon white or red wine
vinegar

1 teaspoon olive oil

Olive oil spray

2 large eggs

Put the lettuce, potato, scallion, and herbs in a bowl. Pour the vinegar and olive oil over the salad and toss gently to combine.

Coat a nonstick skillet with olive oil spray and heat over medium heat. Add the eggs and cook for about 2 minutes, or until the whites are set. Flip the eggs over and slide them onto the salad. Serve.

RATIO (Carb:Protein) = 2:1

PER SERVING: Calories 337 · Protein 13 g · Carbohydrate 28 g · Fiber 5 g · Fat 18 g · Saturated Fat 4 g · Sodium 43 mg

Salmon with Crunchy Vegetables & Celery Root Cream

SERVES 1

This makes enough sauce for four servings, so feel free to scale up the fish and vegetable components and serve this to company.

¼ celery root (celeriac), peeled and quartered

Salt and freshly ground black pepper

Olive oil spray

4 ounces salmon or cod fillet

1 cup mixed vegetables (such as carrot, parsnip, cauliflower, broccoli, and beet), thinly sliced

Chopped mixed fresh herbs, such as parsley, dill, or chervil (optional)

Zest and juice of 1 lemon

1 teaspoon olive oil, for serving

Wildflower honey, for serving

Place the celery root in a saucepan and add water to cover and a pinch of salt. Bring to a boil over high heat and boil for about 18 minutes, or until tender. Drain the celery root, reserving the cooking water. Transfer to a blender and puree, gradually adding about 1 cup of the reserved cooking water, until pureed to a saucelike consistency. Season with salt and pepper.

Meanwhile, coat a nonstick skillet with olive oil and heat over high heat. Add the salmon, skin-side down, and cook for 3 to 4 minutes, or until the skin browns. Flip the salmon, turn off the heat, and let it stand in the skillet for 3 to 4 minutes to continue cooking with the residual pan heat.

Toss the mixed vegetables with the lemon zest and juice. Add the herbs (if using). Transfer the salmon to a plate and add the vegetable mixture. Drizzle with olive oil and honey and serve.

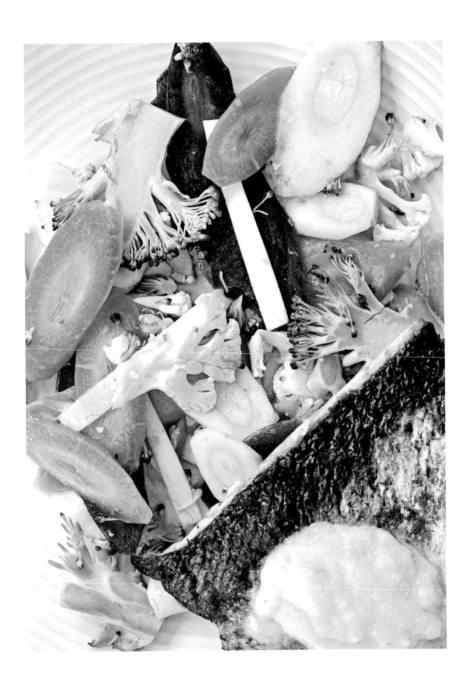

RATIO (Carb:Protein) = 1:1

PER SERVING: Calories 471 • Protein 30 g • Carbohydrate 22 g • Fiber 15 g • Fat 27 g • Saturated Fat 6 g • Sodium 279 mg

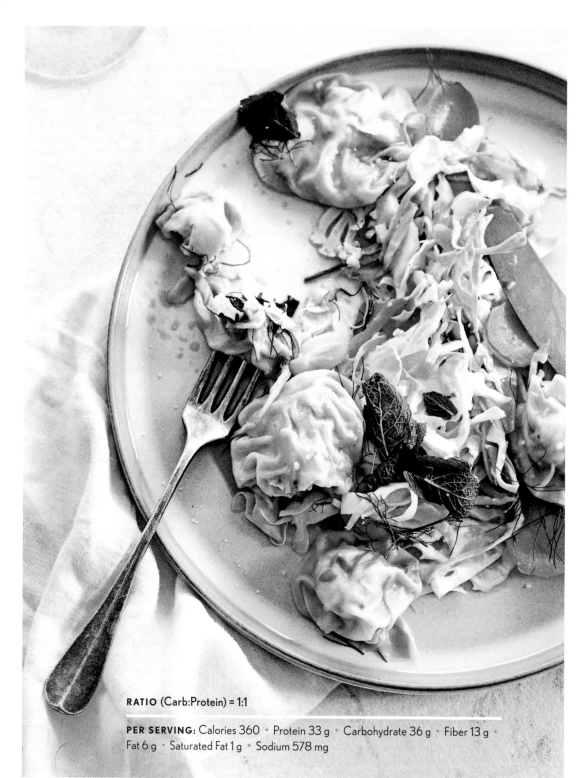

RATIO (Carb:Protein) = 1:1

PER SERVING: Calories 360 • Protein 33 g • Carbohydrate 36 g • Fiber 13 g • Fat 6 g • Saturated Fat 1 g • Sodium 578 mg

Fish Wontons with Cabbage & Carrot Salad

SERVES 1

If you prefer, you can form the fish mixture into two small patties and panfry them; serve on a bed of the shredded vegetables or use them to stuff a low-GI pita.

3½ ounces fish fillet (such as cod or halibut), minced by hand with a sharp knife

⅓ cup small cauliflower florets

⅓ cup small broccoli florets

Salt and freshly ground black pepper

5 wonton wrappers

Handful of mixed fresh herbs, such as parsley and cilantro

¼ green cabbage, cored and shredded

1 small carrot, thinly sliced

1 teaspoon sliced almonds

1 teaspoon soy sauce

Fresh lime juice or lemon juice

Mix the fish, cauliflower, and broccoli in a medium bowl and season with salt and pepper. Divide the mixture among the wonton wrappers. Pull all four corners upward and toward the middle, gently squeeze, and twist the top part to make a small knot.

Place the wontons on a small baking sheet and freeze for 12 minutes.

Bring a medium saucepan of salted water to a boil over high heat. Add the herbs, followed by the wontons. Cook for about 2½ minutes, or until the wontons are golden and have floated to the surface. Use a slotted spoon to transfer to paper towels to drain.

Toss the cabbage, carrot, almonds, and soy sauce in a bowl with lime juice to taste. Add to the wontons and serve.

Fish Fillet
with Radicchio Salad

SERVES 1

A deconstructed tartar sauce brings a tangy counterpoint to this simple breaded fish supper.

1 large egg

Salt and freshly ground black pepper

⅓ cup finely chopped Bircher Muesli (page 87) or store-bought muesli

7 ounces fish fillet, such as cod or halibut

2 teaspoons grapeseed oil

¼ head radicchio

2 cornichons, cut into chunks

Leaves from 6 fresh dill sprigs

2 tablespoons Remoulade (page 212), for serving

Whisk the egg in a shallow bowl with salt and pepper to taste. Place the muesli in a separate shallow bowl. Dip the fish in the egg, allowing any excess egg to drain off. Coat with the muesli.

Heat the oil in a nonstick skillet over medium heat. Add the fish and cook for 3 minutes on each side, or until golden and cooked through. Transfer to a plate.

Toss the radicchio, pickles, and dill together in a medium bowl. Sprinkle over the fish and serve with the remoulade.

RATIO (Carb:Protein) = 1:2

PER SERVING: Calories 330 · Protein 36 g · Carbohydrate 21 g · Fiber 3 g · Fat 12 g · Saturated Fat 5 g · Sodium 676 mg

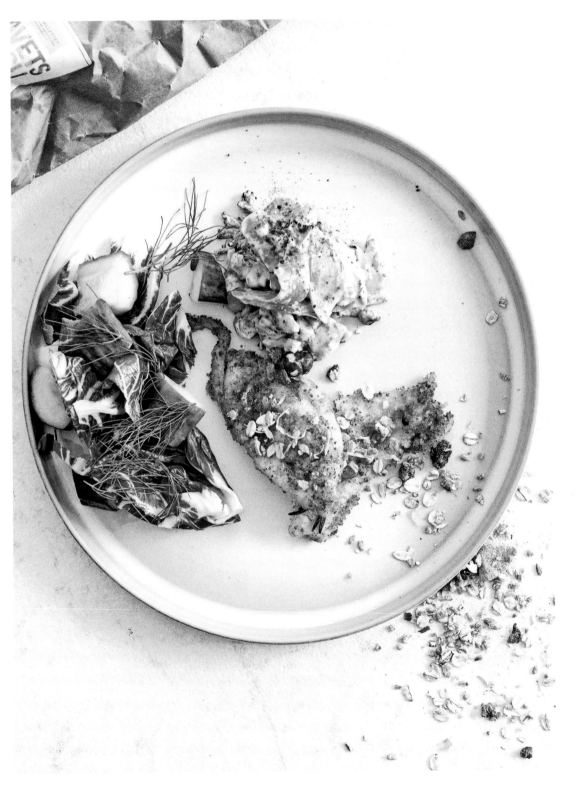

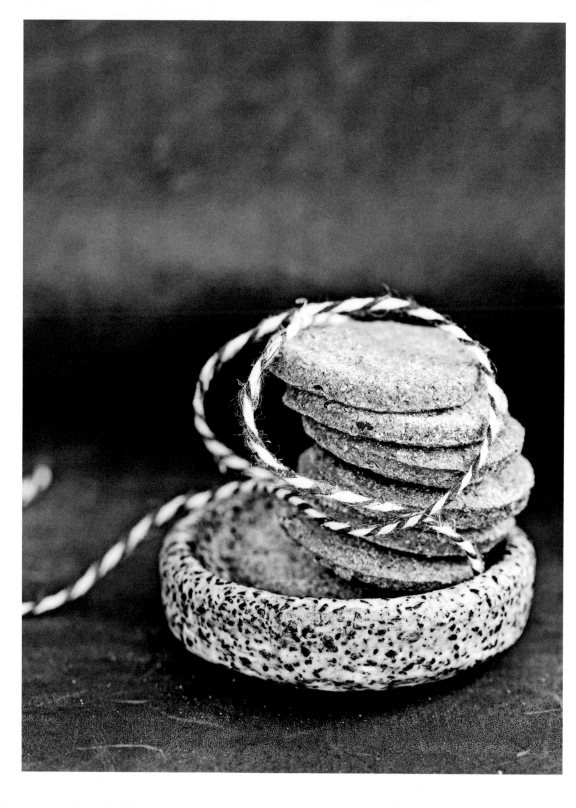

Crispbread

MAKES 18

There is little more than old-fashioned oats and spelt flour in these low-GI crackers, which are easy to make and endlessly useful to have on hand. They will keep for about 2 weeks in an airtight container.

1 cup old-fashioned rolled oats

½ teaspoon salt

2½ cups whole-grain spelt flour, as needed

3 tablespoons canola oil

¼ cup sesame seeds (optional)

Preheat the oven to 350°F. Line two baking sheets with parchment paper.

Combine the oats, salt, and 1½ cups of the flour in the bowl of a stand mixer and beat on medium speed until combined. Mix in the oil. Gradually mix in enough additional spelt flour to make a dough that pulls away from the sides of the bowl. Roll the mixture into 18 equal balls. Place on the prepared baking sheets and press down on each ball with the bottom of a flat glass to flatten them into ⅓-inch-thick discs. Brush with water to glaze and sprinkle with the sesame seeds, if desired. Bake for 15 minutes, or until crisp and golden. Let cool on the baking sheet for 3 minutes, then transfer to a wire rack to cool completely.

RATIO (Carb:Protein) = 4:1

PER SERVING: Calories 122 · Protein 4 g · Carbohydrate 14 g · Fiber 3 g · Fat 5 g · Saturated Fat <1 g · Sodium 128 mg

Avocado-Chocolate Spread

This slightly sweet spread is excellent on low-GI toast or crispbread. Use a good-quality dark chocolate, preferably 72% cacao or more.

3½ ounces bittersweet (at least 70% cacao) chocolate, coarsely chopped

1 ripe avocado, halved and pitted

2 tablespoons sliced natural almonds

1 tablespoon pure wildflower honey

Juice of ½ lime

Salt and freshly ground black pepper

Bring a saucepan filled with about ½ inch of water to a low simmer over low heat. Put the chocolate in a small heatproof bowl, set it over the saucepan (do not let the bottom of the bowl touch the water), and let the chocolate melt, stirring occasionally. Remove the bowl from the pan and let the chocolate cool until tepid.

Scoop the avocado flesh into a food processor and add the chocolate, almonds, honey, and lime juice. Process to a paste and season with salt and pepper.

Transfer to a jar and store in the refrigerator for up to 1 week.

RATIO (Carb:Protein) = 6:1

PER SERVING: Calories 31 · Protein <1 g · Carbohydrate 2 g · Fiber <1 g · Fat 2 g · Saturated Fat 1 g · Sodium 6 mg

Fruit & Nut Spread

MAKES ABOUT 2 CUPS
(2 teaspoons per serving)

Spread sparingly on a crispbread or an apple slice for a midmorning or afternoon energy boost.

6 tablespoons peanut oil

12 dried apricots, diced

5 dried figs, coarsely chopped

¼ cup raisins

10 roasted peanuts

2 tablespoons toasted sliced almonds (see page 99)

1 tablespoon rye berries, toasted in a skillet

1 tablespoon brown sugar

Put the oil, apricots, figs, raisins, peanuts, almonds, rye berries, and brown sugar in a food processor and process until well combined.

Transfer to a jar and store in the refrigerator for up to 3 months.

RATIO (Carb:Protein) = 10:1

PER SERVING (2 TEASPOONS): Calories 46 · Protein <1 g · Carbohydrate 4 g · Fiber 1 g · Fat 3 g · Saturated Fat <1 g · Sodium 33 mg

Whole-Grain Rolls

MAKES ABOUT 20 ROLLS

A blend of grains and seeds make these rolls particularly toothsome. The cooled rolls can be wrapped tightly in plastic, frozen for two to three months, and defrosted as needed.

2 cups warm water
(105° to 115°F)

½ teaspoon instant yeast

1½ cups whole wheat flour

1½ cups spelt flour

2 cups unbleached all-purpose flour, plus more as needed

⅓ cup old-fashioned rolled oats

3 tablespoons hulled sunflower seeds

3 tablespoons toasted unsalted hulled pumpkin seeds (pepitas)

2¼ teaspoons salt

Olive oil for greasing the bowl

Whisk together the water and yeast in a large bowl. Add the whole wheat, spelt, and all-purpose flours, oats, sunflower seeds, pumpkin seeds, and salt and mix well until combined.

Turn the dough out onto a lightly floured work surface. Knead the dough for 8 to 10 minutes, adding more flour if necessary, until it is smooth and elastic. Place in an oiled bowl, cover with a kitchen towel, and let stand in a warm, draft-free place for at least 2 hours, or until almost doubled in volume.

Preheat the oven to 425°F. Line two large baking sheets with parchment paper.

Shape the dough into 20 equal balls. Place on the prepared baking sheets, cover with kitchen towels, and let stand in a warm, draft-free place for about 30 minutes, or until they look slightly puffed. (Or cover the rolls with oiled plastic wrap, oiled-side down, and refrigerate overnight. Let the roll stand at room temperature for about 2 hours to lose their chill before baking.)

Bake the rolls for 20 minutes, or until they are golden and sound hollow when tapped on the bottom. Transfer to wire racks and let cool.

RATIO (Carb:Protein) = 5:1 Per Roll

PER SERVING: Calories 134 · Protein 5 g · Carbohydrate 23 g · Fiber 3 g · Fat 2 g · Saturated Fat <1 g · Sodium 192 mg

Hummus

Homemade hummus is your secret weapon for adding filling protein and creamy texture to so many next-to-instant meals. Try the variations (see opposite) when you want to change it up.

1 cup dried chickpeas

¼ cup canola oil

1 hot green chile, such as jalapeño or serrano, seeded and minced

2 teaspoons ground cumin

1 teaspoon finely grated fresh ginger

1 garlic clove, finely chopped

Salt and freshly ground black pepper

The day before making the hummus, put the chickpeas in a bowl, cover with plenty of cold water, and refrigerate overnight.

Drain the chickpeas; rinse well. Discard any discolored chickpeas. Place the chickpeas in a large saucepan, cover with at least 1 inch of water, and bring to a boil over medium-high heat. Reduce the heat to medium and simmer briskly for 20 to 30 minutes, until the chickpeas are tender (timing will depend on the dryness of the beans). Scoop out and reserve 1¼ cups of the cooking water. Drain and rinse the chickpeas. Let them cool.

Combine the chickpeas, oil, lemon juice, chile, cumin, ginger, and garlic in a food processor. Process until well blended. With the motor running, gradually enough of the reserved cooking water to reach the desired texture, being careful not to make it too thin to allow for seasoning. Season with lemon juice, salt, and pepper.

Variations

KIDNEY BEAN AND BEET HUMMUS: Substitute dried kidney beans for the chickpeas. Before processing, add ½ cup coarsely chopped roasted or boiled beet and a small handful of fresh parsley.

WHITE BEAN AND PARMESAN HUMMUS: Substitute dried white beans (cannellini) for the chickpeas. Before processing, add 1 cup freshly grated Parmesan cheese and a pinch of dried oregano.

LENTIL AND SUN-DRIED TOMATO HUMMUS: Omit the chickpeas. Cook 2 cups dried green lentils in plenty of boiling water for 20 minutes, or until tender. Drain and rinse. Before processing, add ½ cup drained oil-packed sun-dried tomatoes and 10 fresh basil leaves.

RATIO (Carb:Protein) = 2:1

PER SERVING (½ CUP): Calories 161 · Protein 4 g · Carbohydrate 28 g · Fiber 4 g · Fat 3 g · Saturated Fat 2 g · Sodium 30 mg

Baked Strawberry Jam

The flavor of licorice is very popular in Scandinavia; it adds an elusive but delicious note to this preserve.

9 ounces strawberries, hulled but left whole

2 tablespoons sugar

2 tablespoons wildflower honey

1 teaspoon ground cinnamon

2 star anise pods

Zest and juice of 1 lemon

1 teaspoon powdered licorice root (optional)

Preheat the oven to 350°F. Line a baking sheet with parchment paper.

Combine the strawberries, sugar, honey, cinnamon, anise, lemon zest, lemon juice, and licorice (if using) in a large bowl. Scrape onto the prepared baking sheet. Bake for 15 minutes, or until the berries are soft.

Return to the bowl. Discard the star anise and stir the jam well until combined. Pour into a hot, sterilized 1½-cup jar. Let cool, uncovered. Cover the jar and store in the refrigerator for up to 2 weeks.

PER SERVING (1 TABLESPOON): Calories 22 · Protein <1 g · Carbohydrate 5 g · Fiber 1 g · Fat <1 g · Saturated Fat <1 g · Sodium 2 mg

Basic Yogurt Dip

This dip and the variations that follow are ideal for quick snacks; keep one or several on hand so you'll never have to forage for a healthy bite to tide you over between meals.

⅔ cup low-fat Greek yogurt

1 tablespoon wildflower honey

1 tablespoon Dijon mustard

1 tablespoon fresh lime juice

Salt and freshly ground black pepper

Mix the yogurt, honey, mustard, and lime juice in a medium bowl. Season with salt and pepper.

Variations

CURRY AND APPLE: Add ½ chopped apple, 1 tablespoon curry powder, and 1 tablespoon chopped mango chutney.

SWEET CHILI: Add 2 tablespoons Thai sweet chili sauce and 1 finely chopped garlic clove.

MIXED HERB: Add a handful of chopped mixed fresh herbs, such as dill, chives, and fresh chopped parsley leaves.

TARTARE: Add 2 tablespoons chopped cornichons, 1 tablespoon rinsed nonpareil capers, 1 tablespoon finely chopped red onion, and 1 tablespoon chopped fresh parsley.

RAITA: Add 2 tablespoons chopped almonds, ¼ finely chopped seedless (English) cucumber, 2 tablespoons thinly sliced fresh mint, and ½ minced garlic clove.

RATIO (Carb:Protein) = 2:0

PER SERVING: Calories 161 · Protein 4 g · Carbohydrate 28 g · Fiber 4 g · Fat 3 g · Saturated Fat 2 g · Sodium 30 mg

Salad Dressing

This is perfect for raw vegetables.

3 tablespoons Dijon mustard

3 tablespoons apple juice

⅓ cup plus 2 tablespoons white wine vinegar

⅓ cup plus 2 tablespoons canola oil

Whisk the mustard, apple juice, and vinegar in a medium bowl. Gradually whisk in the oil.

PER SERVING (1 TABLESPOON): Calories 60 · Protein <1 g · Carbohydrate <1 g · Fiber <1 g · Fat 6 g · Saturated Fat <1 g · Sodium 63.1 mg

Roasted Red Pepper Sauce

MAKES ABOUT 2 CUPS

Vegetable oil, for the baking sheet

3 red bell peppers, halved and seeded

1 shallot, finely chopped

⅓ cup plus 2 tablespoons red wine vinegar

2 tablespoons pure wildflower honey

1 small fennel bulb, outer layer removed, finely diced

2 teaspoons fresh oregano leaves, or 1 teaspoon dried oregano

1 sprig lovage or celery frond, leaves chopped

Preheat the oven to 500°F. Line a baking sheet with aluminum foil and coat lightly with oil.

Place the bell peppers on the prepared baking sheet, skin-side up. Roast for about 15 minutes, until the skin blisters and blackens. Transfer to a heatproof bowl, cover with plastic wrap, and let stand for 15 minutes. Peel and seed the peppers. Dice the flesh, reserving any juices.

Bring the shallot, vinegar, and honey to a boil in a small saucepan over medium heat. Cook for 2 to 3 minutes, or until slightly reduced. Add the fennel, oregano, and lovage, with any pepper juices. Bring to a simmer and cook for about 5 minutes, or until the fennel is crisp-tender. Transfer to a bowl.

Stir in the chopped red bell pepper and let cool to room temperature. Serve with meat or fish.

PER SERVING (1½ TABLESPOONS): Calories 18 · Protein <1 g · Carbohydrate 3 g · Fiber 1 g · Fat <1 g · Saturated Fat (g) <1 g · Sodium (mg) 5 mg

Remoulade

MAKES ABOUT 2 CUPS

½ cup low-fat plain skyr or
   Cheater's Skyr (page 231)
1 tablespoon Dijon mustard
2 tablespoons fresh lemon juice
1 tablespoon curry powder

1 cup chopped or sliced
   seasonal vegetables, such
   as cauliflower, carrots, and
   onions
2 sour pickles, sliced
Salt and freshly ground black
   pepper

Mix the skyr, mustard, lemon juice, and curry powder in a medium bowl. Stir in the vegetables and pickles. Season with salt and pepper.

PER SERVING (¼ CUP): Calories 36 · Protein 3 g · Carbohydrate 5 g · Fiber 2 g · Fat <1 g · Saturated Fat <1 g · Sodium 102 mg

Sweet-and-Sour Sauce

MAKES 4 TABLESPOONS

2 tablespoons tomato ketchup

1 tablespoon no-sugar-added blueberry or blackberry syrup

1 tablespoon pure wildflower honey

1 teaspoon Worcestershire sauce

3 drops hot sauce

Whisk the ketchup, syrup, honey, Worcestershire sauce, and hot sauce in a small bowl.

PER SERVING (1 TABLESPOON): Calories 30 · Protein <1 g · Carbohydrate 8 g · Fiber <1 g · Fat <1 g · Saturated Fat <1 g · Sodium 94 mg

Red Wine, Mustard & Herb Sauce

2 teaspoons olive oil

1 shallot, finely chopped

2 tablespoons red wine vinegar

¾ cup plus 2 tablespoons
hearty red wine

½ cup chicken or vegetable
stock

1 tablespoon Dijon mustard

6 sprigs fresh thyme

3 bay leaves

2 teaspoons unsalted butter or
heavy cream (optional)

Pinch of sugar

Salt and freshly ground white
pepper

Heat the olive oil in a medium saucepan over medium heat. Add the shallot
and cook, stirring often, for 2 to 3 minutes, or until softened. Add the vinegar
and reduce the heat to low. Simmer, stirring often, for 5 minutes, or until the
vinegar has reduced by half.

Add the wine, stock, mustard, thyme, and bay leaves and simmer over
medium-low heat, stirring occasionally, for 10 minutes to blend the flavors.

Remove from the heat. Whisk in the butter (if using) and the sugar. If you
have any pan juices from a roast or sauté, add them to the sauce. Season with
salt and white pepper. Strain the sauce through a fine-mesh sieve into a sauce-
boat or medium bowl. Serve warm.

PER 100 ML (WITH BUTTER): Calories 350 · Protein 5 g · Carbohydrate 12 g ·
Fiber 7 g · Fat 20 g · Saturated Fat 8 g · Sodium 923 mg

Spicy Mint Marinade

MAKES ABOUT 7/8 CUP

1 orange

2 tablespoons red wine vinegar

2 tablespoons finely chopped
fresh mint

1 tablespoon pure wildflower
honey

2 teaspoons toasted sesame oil

6 thin slices hot green chile,
such as jalapeño

Remove half the orange zest in strips with a vegetable peeler. Juice the orange.

Whisk the orange zest, orange juice, vinegar mint, honey, sesame oil, and chile together in a small bowl. Use as a marinade for beef, chicken, pork, or lamb.

PER SERVING (2 TABLESPOONS): Calories 220 · Protein 1 g · Carbohydrate 31 g · Fiber 3 g · Fat 9 g · Saturated Fat 1 g · Sodium 14 mg

Pickled Vegetables

MAKES ABOUT 5½ CUPS

4½ cups apple cider vinegar

⅔ cup apple juice

⅔ cup sugar

1 teaspoon yellow mustard seeds

4 bay leaves

1 tablespoon salt

1 teaspoon whole black peppercorns

About 4 cups assorted seasonal vegetables, such as cauliflower florets, carrot rounds or sticks, zucchini (or yellow squash) rounds or sticks, kirby cucumber rounds or sticks, and/or seeded red bell pepper sticks

Bring the vinegar, apple juice, sugar, mustard seeds, bay leaves, salt, and pepper to a boil in a medium nonreactive saucepan over high heat.

Place the vegetables in a large heatproof bowl. Pour over enough hot pickling liquid to cover the vegetables. Let cool. Transfer the vegetables and liquid to hot sterilized jars with lids, seal, and refrigerate. The pickled vegetables can be stored in the refrigerator for up to 1 month. These make a great snack or accompaniment to many dishes.

PER 100 G: Calories 118 • Protein 2 g • Carbohydrate 21 g • Fiber 2 g • Fat 1 g • Saturated Fat <1 g • Sodium 220 mg

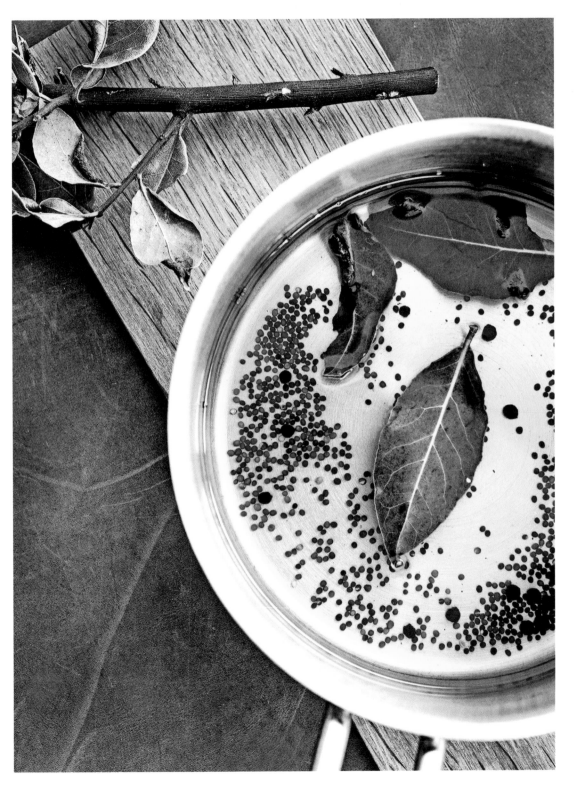

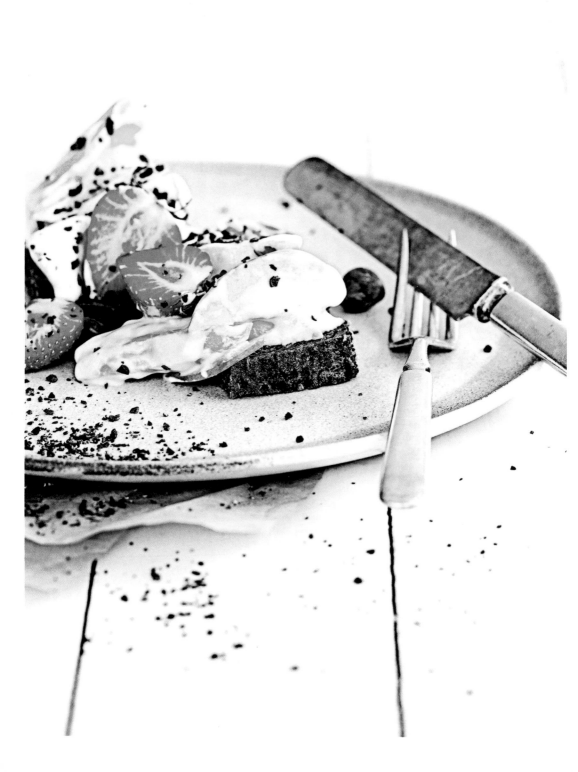

Honey Bruschetta

SERVES 2

When you don't have time to make a dessert, assemble these pretty, sweet toasts from pantry ingredients.

1 teaspoon pure wildflower honey

2 slices whole-grain rye bread or whole rye pumpernickel bread, toasted

¼ cup low-fat plain skyr or Cheater's Skyr (page 231)

1 teaspoon confectioners' sugar

1 cup mixed seasonal fruit, cut into bite-size pieces

1 tablespoon chopped toasted almonds, walnuts, or hazelnuts (see pages 99 and 80)

1 teaspoon finely chopped bittersweet chocolate (about 70% cacao)

Spread the honey over the bread.

Mix the skyr and confectioners' sugar together in a medium bowl. Fold in the fruit.

Spoon the fruit mixture over the bread. Sprinkle with the nuts and chocolate. Serve.

RATIO (Carb:Protein) = 4:1

PER SERVING: Calories 191 · Protein 7 g · Carbohydrate 28 g · Fiber 4 g · Fat 5 g · Saturated Fat 1 g · Sodium 239 mg

Cherry Compote with Vanilla Ricotta

SERVES 1

With a dish this simple, it's important to choose the best ingredients you can find. Searching out fresh ricotta cheese is well worth the effort. This would also work as a weekend breakfast.

8 fresh cherries, pitted and halved

2 tablespoons unsweetened cranberry juice

1 teaspoon pure wildflower honey

⅓ cup fresh low-fat ricotta

¼ teaspoon pure vanilla extract

Bring the cherries, cranberry juice, and ½ teaspoon of the honey to a simmer in a small saucepan over medium heat. Simmer, stirring occasionally, for 3 to 4 minutes, or until the cherries are plump and syrupy. Let cool.

Stir the ricotta, remaining ½ teaspoon honey, and the vanilla together in a small bowl. Transfer to a jar or bowl, top with the cherry compote, and serve.

RATIO (Carb:Protein) = 2:1

PER SERVING: Calories 168 · Protein 10 g · Carbohydrate 20 g · Fiber 1 g · Fat 5 g · Saturated Fat 3 g · Sodium 179 mg

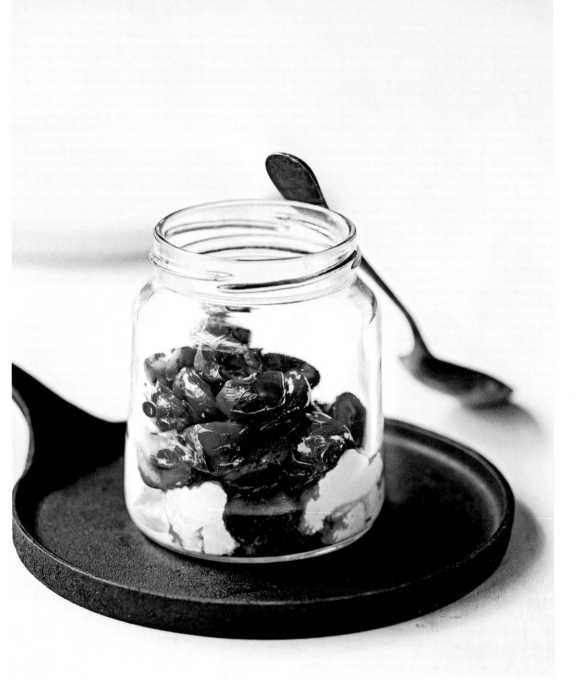

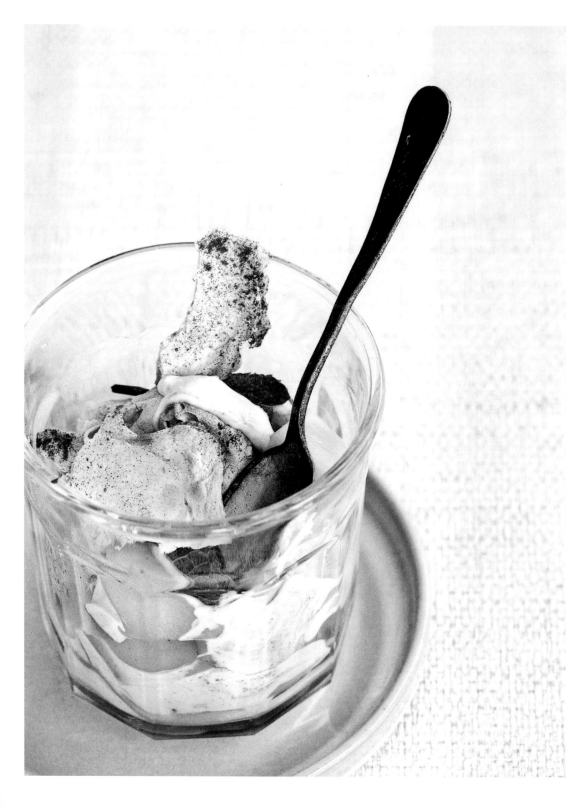

Trifle with
Mango, Meringues & Skyr

SERVES 1

Traditional trifle is made with soaked cake pieces; our version substitutes crushed meringue cookies, resulting in a lighter dessert that won't weigh you down.

2 tablespoons low-fat plain skyr or Cheater's Skyr (page 231)

1 teaspoon pure wildflower honey, plus more for serving

2 store-bought meringue cookies, crushed

¼ mango or other seasonal fruit, diced

4 to 6 fresh mint leaves

Fresh lime juice, for serving

Mix the skyr with the honey.

Layer the skyr mixture, crushed meringues, mango, and mint leaves in a glass, alternating the ingredients as you build up the trifle. Drizzle with lime juice and extra honey, and serve.

RATIO (Carb:Protein) = 7:1

PER SERVING: Calories 182 · Protein 5 g · Carbohydrate 39 g · Fiber 2 g · Fat 1 g · Saturated Fat 0 g · Sodium 15 mg

Whole Orange &
Almond Yogurt Cake

SERVES 12

While not entirely gluten-free due to a small amount of flour in the batter, this cake is based on ricotta cheese, dairy, and almond meal, which accounts for both its moist, rich texture and low-GI rating.

4 small navel oranges

Vegetable oil for greasing the pan

⅔ cup fresh low-fat ricotta

½ cup low-GI sugar, such as coconut palm or maple sugar

2 large eggs

1½ cups almond flour or almond meal

½ cup self-rising flour

1 teaspoon baking powder

2 cups fat-free Greek yogurt

Confectioners' sugar, for serving

Place 2 of the whole oranges in a large saucepan, add cold water to cover, and bring to a boil over high heat. Drain, cover with fresh water, and return to a boil. Reduce the heat to low and simmer for 1 hour, adding more water if needed. Drain well and let cool completely.

Preheat the oven to 300°F. Lightly grease a 9-inch round cake pan and line the bottom and sides with parchment paper.

Cut the cooled oranges into quarters, discarding the seeds. Process the orange quarters and ricotta in a food processor until smooth. Put the sugar and eggs in a large bowl and beat with an electric mixer on high speed until thick and pale, about 3 minutes. Fold in the orange mixture. Add the almond flour, self-rising flour, baking powder, and ½ cup of the yogurt and stir until well combined.

Spoon the batter into the prepared pan. Bake for 1 hour 10 minutes, or until a wooden skewer inserted into the center comes out with a few moist crumbs clinging to it. Cover the top of the cake with aluminum foil if it is browning too quickly. Let cool on a wire rack for 20 minutes. Carefully invert and unmold the cake onto a plate, transfer, right-side up, to a wire rack, and let cool completely.

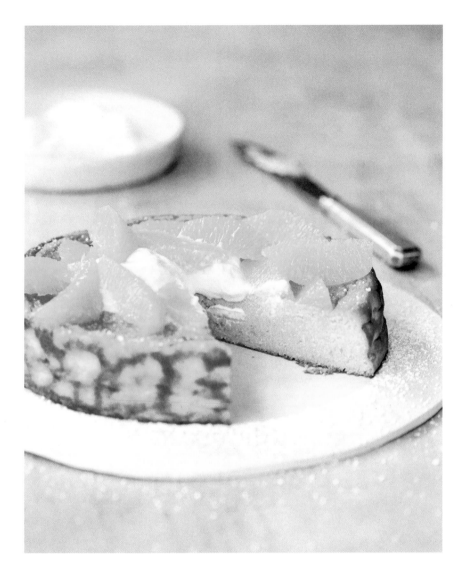

Meanwhile, peel and segment the remaining oranges. Dust the top of the cake with confectioners' sugar. Slice and serve each portion with the orange segments and a dollop of the remaining yogurt.

RATIO (Carb:Protein) = 2:1

PER SERVING: Calories 200 · Protein 10 g · Carbohydrate 17 g · Fiber 3 g · Fat 9 g · Saturated Fat 2 g · Sodium 241 mg

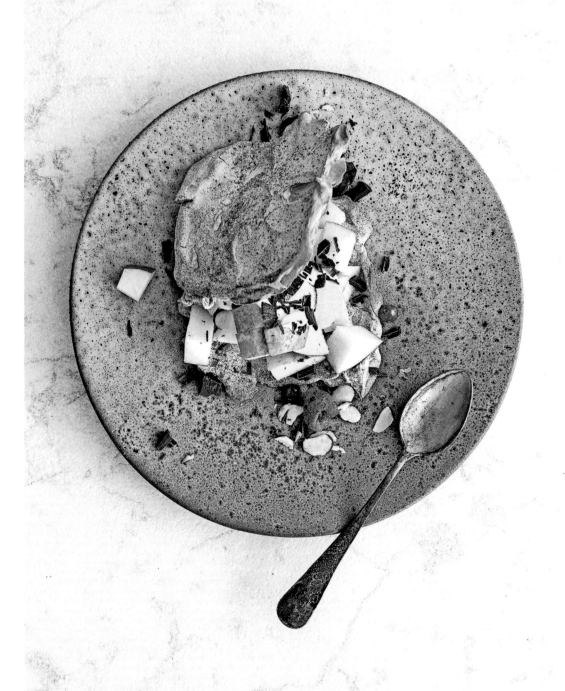

Meringues with Chocolate & Fruit Skyr

SERVES 4

Protein-rich skyr rather than sweetened whipped cream tops these mini pavlovas, which make an elegant base for fruit, nuts, and a touch of chocolate.

2 large egg whites, at room temperature

½ cup superfine sugar

1 cup low-fat plain skyr or Cheater's Skyr (page 231)

2 apples, cored and diced

2 pears, cored and diced

¼ cup raspberries, blueberries, or red currants

¼ cup sliced or finely chopped almonds

2 ounces bittersweet (about 70% cacao) chocolate, finely chopped

Preheat the oven to 250°F. Line two large baking sheets with parchment paper.

Whip the egg whites in a clean, dry bowl with an electric mixer on high speed until they hold stiff peaks. Gradually beat in the sugar, 1 tablespoon at a time, and whip until the mixture holds very stiff, shiny peaks and the sugar has completely dissolved.

Spoon the mixture onto the baking sheets in four wide rounds, 1½ to 2 inches thick. Bake the meringues for 1½ hours, or until crisp and lightly browned.

Place each meringue on its own plate. Top with equal amounts of the skyr, apples, pears, raspberries, almonds, and chocolate.

RATIO (Carb:Protein) = 6:1

PER SERVING: Calories 510 · Protein 14 g · Carbohydrate 89 g · Fiber 7 g · Fat 11 g · Saturated Fat 3 g · Sodium 57 mg

Caramelized Pineapple & Strawberries with Cardamom Custard

Cardamom is a warm spice frequently found in Scandinavian baked goods. Here it is used to scent a simple custard served with caramelized fruits.

1¼ cups low-fat milk

1 teaspoon pure vanilla extract

¼ teaspoon ground cardamom

2 large eggs

1 tablespoon plus 1 teaspoon low-GI sugar, such as coconut palm or maple sugar

1½ teaspoons cornstarch

4 thin slices pineapple (about 5 ounces total)

Scant 1 cup sliced strawberries

1 tablespoon toasted hulled pumpkins seeds (pepitas), for serving

Bring the milk, vanilla, and cardamom to a simmer in a small saucepan over medium heat. Remove from the heat.

Whisk the eggs, 1 tablespoon of the sugar, and the cornstarch well in a medium bowl until pale. While whisking continuously, gradually pour in the hot milk mixture. Return this mixture to a rinsed-out saucepan and stir over low heat until the custard thickens and coats the back of a spoon (your finger, drawn through the custard, will cut a swath). Do not allow the custard to boil. Pour the custard through a fine-mesh sieve into a small bowl. Cover with plastic wrap pressed directly against the surface to prevent a skin from forming. If desired, let cool completely, then refrigerate for at least 2 hours, or until chilled.

Toss the pineapple, strawberries, and remaining 1 teaspoon sugar in a medium bowl. Heat a large nonstick skillet over high heat. Add the fruit and cook, stirring occasionally, for 2 to 3 minutes, or until lightly caramelized. Transfer to serving dishes and sprinkle with the pumpkin seeds. Serve hot with the warm (or chilled) custard.

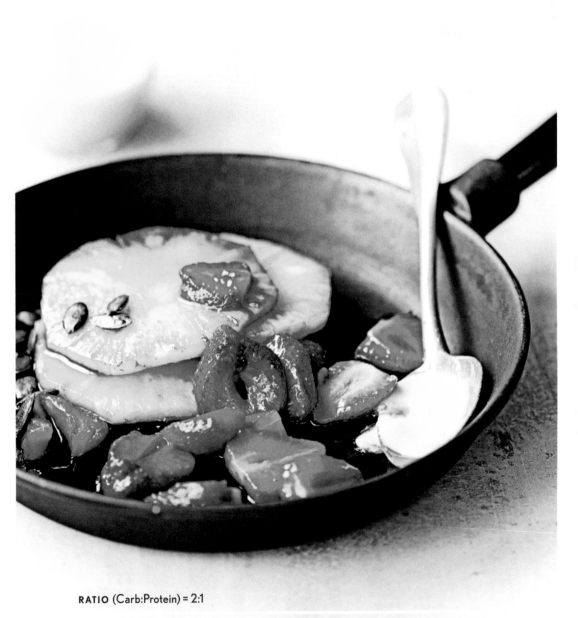

RATIO (Carb:Protein) = 2:1

PER SERVING: Calories 256 • Protein 15 g • Carbohydrate 27 g • Fiber 3 g • Fat 9 g • Saturated Fat 2 g • Sodium 129 mg

Homemade Granola

SERVES 20 (¼ cup per serving)

Our signature granola reverses the typical grain-to-nut balance for a blend that has a bit more protein than what you get at the store—as well as a somewhat higher fat content (although it is healthy unsaturated fat).

1 cup raw whole almonds

1 cup skinned toasted hazelnuts (see page 80)

½ cup raw unsalted hulled pumpkin seeds (pepitas)

⅔ cup old-fashioned rolled oats or barley flakes

⅔ cup rolled rye flakes or additional rolled oats

⅓ cup pure wildflower honey

2 tablespoons light brown sugar

⅞ cup sweetened dried cranberries or dried blueberries

1 tablespoon chia seeds

Preheat the oven to 425°F. Line a baking sheet with parchment paper.

Spread the almonds, hazelnuts, pepitas, oats, and rye flakes over the prepared baking sheet and bake for 10 minutes. Remove from the oven. Drizzle with the honey and sprinkle with the sugar. Add the cranberries and chia seeds and mix well. Return to the oven and bake for 5 minutes more, or until the granola is lightly browned.

Let cool completely. Store the granola in an airtight container at room temperature.

RATIO (Carb:Protein) = 4:1

PER SERVING (¼ CUP): Calories 150 · Protein 4 g · Carbohydrate 15 g · Fiber 2 g · Fat 8 g · Saturated Fat 1 g · Sodium 3 mg

Cheater's Skyr

Skyr has been part of the Scandinavian diet for millennia, and the rest of the world is now taking note of its rich flavor and probiotic qualities. It is similar to *labneh* in that it can be served as a spread on its own, as a flavored topping, or like yogurt. You may be able to purchase authentic skyr in your local market; if not, this is a good stand-in.

2 cups low-fat Greek yogurt

Line a fine-mesh sieve with a piece of cheesecloth and set it over a bowl. Spoon the yogurt into the sieve, fold the cheesecloth over to cover to yogurt, and refrigerate the setup overnight to drain. Transfer the drained yogurt to an airtight container and store in the refrigerator. It should keep as long as the expiration date on the yogurt container.

RATIO (Carb:Protein) = 1:8

PER SERVING (1 CUP): Calories 200 · Protein 38 g · Carbohydrate 5 g · Fiber 0 g · Fat 2 g · Saturated Fat 2 g · Sodium 25 mg

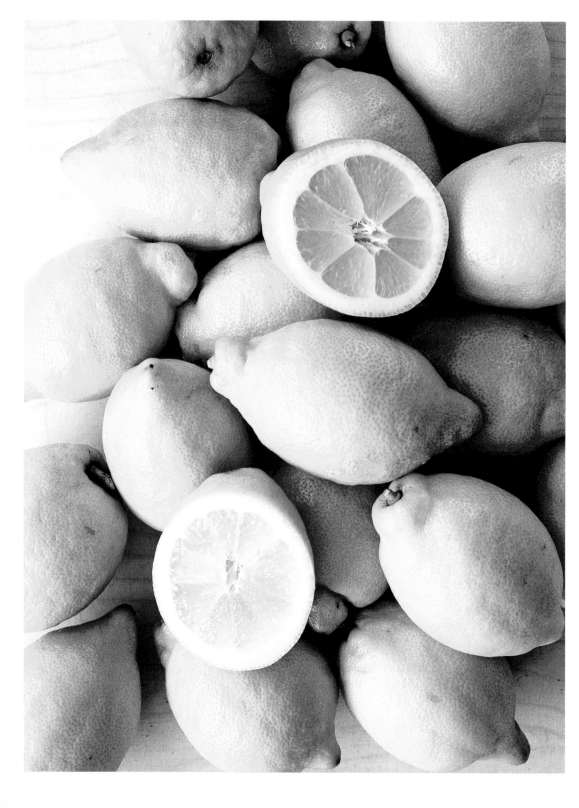

INDEX

Page numbers in *italics* refer to photos.